Other books by David Davies:

The Rice Bowl of Asia

Journey into the Stone Age

*The Influence of Teeth, Diet and
Habits on the Human Face*

A Dictionary of Anthropology

The Centenarians
of the Andes

The Centenarians
of the Andes

DAVID DAVIES

Anchor Press/Doubleday
Garden City, New York
1975

This book was originally published in England by Barrie and
Jenkins, Ltd., 1975.

ISBN: 0-385-09914-2
LIBRARY OF CONGRESS CATALOG CARD NUMBER 75-6270
COPYRIGHT © 1975 DAVID DAVIES
ALL RIGHTS RESERVED
PRINTED IN THE UNITED STATES OF AMERICA
FIRST EDITION IN THE UNITED STATES OF AMERICA

CONTENTS

PREFACE

This book describes the four visits that I made over a period of three years to Vilcabamba and the surrounding areas of southern Ecuador between 1971 and the end of 1973, the studies carried out on these visits, and their results.

On the first and the last of the visits I was alone; for two I was accompanied by my wife. While visiting the area in May–July 1973, the local Department of Public Health, under Dr. Hugo Gonzalez, kindly loaned me Dr. Lolita Samaniego and a nurse. They were invaluable for the three hundred or so interviews that I carried out, on a cross section of the community. With the centenarians Dr. Samaniego was especially popular as she was gay and cheerful and always ready to joke. I was particularly grateful for her help, as the centenarians had never had anything like an interview experience before. During this time Mr. Michael Fuller acted as technician and photographer. He took some two thousand photographs and a film. We also had the services of Alberto Donadio, a conservationist, from the University of the Andes in Colombia, who joined us from time to time.

The rector of Loja University supplied us with a jeep and students for assistance when required, when we went to the remote villages. For visits to Vilcabamba only it was the Department of Public Health that loaned us a jeep. In order to visit the regions away from the tracks, Indian-type ponies and shanks' pony were also used.

I was able to go to South America because the Winston Churchill Memorial Trust had awarded me a grant for the study of human ecology in Colombia and Ecuador.

While in Quito in March 1971, the Ecuadoran Department of External Affairs gave us the names of scientists in the field of human ecology whom it would be useful to contact. This we did, learning from them of some interesting people to be found at Vilcabamba; therefore the knowledge of that place is not really new. However, the discovery of the other villages, and the crescent with its groups of people who are even older than those to be found in Vilcabamba, is entirely new and makes the whole area of much more importance.

It also suggests that whatever it is that makes these villages conducive to longevity might, one day, be applied to the rest of mankind, if the sites can be preserved long enough for scientific study. So the Vilcabambans have been raised in status from a group of genetic fossils toward an applied immortality—that which everyone is seeking either consciously or subconsciously.

I was asked to prepare plans for a sanitorium for Vilcabamba, but as I was only beginning at that time to discover the true extent of the area I did not submit anything, as I feel that something far more embracing is required: e.g. a sanitorium and a laboratory, combined. At the sanitorium, some of the centenarians could be studied, and specially selected outsiders could stay to see what effect the environment had upon them. At the laboratories the fauna and the flora could be studied in detail, and the diet, as well as blood samples, could be studied on the spot: this would prevent them from deteriorating during travel. It goes without saying that no research would be unnecessarily duplicated.

I would suggest that Loja should be the center for administration, and a record kept of all the studies made by scientists and doctors who visit.

Ecuador is rapidly becoming a wealthy nation, and a time will come when she will take a look at her natural assets, which are many, and I'm sure that these centenarians will be included. It is to the advantage of world science that we retain this area for posterity.

Our team consisted of Alberto Donadio, a Colombian scientist from the University of the Andes; Michael Fuller from London, who was our technician and photographer; Dr. Lolita Samaniego and her nurse from Loja, Mariela Sarongo; Magdalena Reyes, a social scientist from Loja; Patrice Sauman from Quito; a dentist, Dr. Hector Fabara and Numa Reinoso, a lecturer from the University in Loja.

INTRODUCTION

The population explosion continues and countries become increasingly overcrowded. Anything in a minority, out of the ordinary or not geared to the life of the majority, be it fauna, flora or minority groups, must inevitably suffer. Innumerable species of plants and animals have become extinct during the last hundred years. So have some groups of people: in the Americas, many tribes of plains Indians, and the Yagans of Tierra del Fuego; in Australia, the Tasmanians. These are only three of many examples.

Only recently has concern, largely futile, been felt for the disappearance of peoples living more "primitive" ways of life. But I feel that a plea—at least from the medical point of view—should be made for them. These people, who often live in continuous close contact with nature, have much to offer us in their way of life. Our lives have become far removed from the natural elements, and in cutting ourselves off we have lost much that is valuable.

From these tribes we gain and have gained many invaluable cures for illnesses. For instance, the curare poison, found to be an unsurpassed heart stimulant, was found, under great difficulties, by a British doctor. For many years the only known antidote to malaria was quinine, or, as it was called in days gone by "Peruvian bark." This bark was first used among the Indians only twenty miles from Vilcabamba, the first village we discovered in Ecuador. This village was found to have people living to a remarkably old age.

This brings me to the main purpose of this book, which is to present the first study of the oldest authenticated living people to be found in the world today. These people live in a number of villages in southern Ecuador. Until recently, the most noted of these was Vilcabamba, although now we have found centenarians living in a whole arc of villages in the area. These people have been more or less ignored by the medical profession although investigating them requires little funding.

Some scientists now hold that the environment may be just as important a factor in aging as genetics. Most scientists have considered genetics one of the holiest of holy cows. They have concentrated on experiments on animals and cellular structure activity, and have seen in environmental studies a threat. But the people in Ecuador, some living to the age of 140 years or more, must be studied immediately—it does not require years of experiments upon animals which might eventually lead to the first tentative studies upon humans.

Studies in gerontology, prevention of aging, can only be helped by looking at the whole person in the aging process. Without this, the actual conditions of life which might allow people to live longer cannot be assessed. The old people of Ecuador provide a marvelous opportunity to explore the possible environmental factors that slow down the aging process. They are thus a most exciting and important discovery. Not only do they live to remarkable ages, but they retain their faculties and good health to an extraordinary extent.

Sadly, many sources of knowledge and information have been grossly neglected. The medical profession, being naturally conservative, is suspicious of gaining knowledge from the manuals of local medicine men and witch doctors. But with the rapid disappearance of "primitive" man, some possibly valuable preventatives and cures may also be lost. Time is getting short for exploring these possibilities. Unfortunately such communities are often surrounded by the ignorant, and they are often explored by people with interests other than investigating their way of life. Sadly, too, these people often have the greatest say and influence in their dispersal, and disposal.

There is an increasing feeling in the more technologically advanced areas of the world that people are dissatisfied with the pressures and tensions of life, and with often poor health. The more people know, the more aware they are of what they do not know. Diet and the food factor in our lives and health is a question concerning many people but in some respects this is an area where we are still living in the Victorian era. This is thrown into even sharper relief by the vast improvements in technological fields. It is in communities where people live a life often of extreme simplicity that some of the dietary and living conditions most conducive to health can be seen. It is imperative that these factors are explored.

People have always felt some desire for immortality, and certainly the possibilities of living to an old age have vastly increased in the last fifty years. However, no one wants to live a long life with their faculties impaired.

Very few people think far ahead into their old age to consider all the complications that might arise; very few take steps to retain their health and faculties. Such a change of attitude would affect population size, but also, importantly, our attitudes to the old would have to change radically. We would have to rethink our ideas on retirement, and the role of the aged in communities and families.

But over all, there would have to be a better understanding of ourselves, for this whole sphere of man's existence is being, and has been, neglected. We know a lot about the body; we are told much about our sexual lives; the clergy can also tell us where we go in the end. But in the area of the actual gears of life—what makes us tick, and tick well, and what makes the ticking stop—we know very little. The subject has been terribly neglected. We know little of why in some people cell life and cell renewal continues for much longer than in others.

Apart from the people of Vilcabamba, with its remarkable arc of attendant villages, the Hunzas, and the Russian Abkhasian groups, there are also those old people whom we all meet from time to time who as individuals look, and physically are, remarkably young for their ages. We don't know why. Some of it may be to do with genes, but there are certainly other factors at work—environmental ones, which we are now beginning to investigate. Some occupations attract certain diseases, and others attract longevity (for instance, farm workers and clergymen). Some people are convinced that their diet helps them remain vigorous and healthy for longer.

A genetic approach to aging is entirely different from the environmental approach. Much more work and money have been spent on the former; the latter is only in its infancy, for it is only recently that people living to a very active and healthy old age have been known to exist. There is much prejudice about their study, and few scientists are trained for it.

It seems that those people who have the best chance of a healthy and active old age are those who use their minds and bodies much, even toward the end of their life span. This is certainly true of the centenarians in southern Ecuador. These people also have a lot of sleep. The people who seem to live the shortest lives are those who try in many ways to conserve their energy and their powers, using their brains and little else, and living a very sedentary life. Lawyers and academics often die fairly young.

This book has, therefore, two facets. It is a straightforward study of people remarkable for their healthy longevity. But, at the same time, it is a plea that all peoples set apart from twentieth-century civilization should be more highly regarded and a greater value set on what they can teach us. We can apply their acquired knowledge to our own civilization, even though they may make an apparently humble contribution to our way of life. These Ecuadorans give us a whiff of immortality. We should explore it further. The following factors were the ones we studied—some obviously much more significant than others, alone or in combination: some form of genetic factor; tranquillity in the way of life in the valleys and the lack of stress, due to being isolated; the temperature, for the temperature remains very even in all these places, at an average of 19° Centigrade at midday; the dry climate, apparent in all these areas for most of the year; some elements in the water and soil; some element in the diet—the greatest ages were found in the areas where people lived on a subsistence diet, and one very low in calories; lack of animal fats; altitude; race; some form of medicinal herbs; and the fact that the whole of the region lies close to the Equator (this factor might affect other groups, such as those in southern Arabia). The following account shows the results of our inquiries.

The Centenarians
of the Andes

1
Cultural Attitudes
to the Old

Industrialized societies traditionally have not felt the same deep concern and respect for the aged as non-industrialized, so-called less developed societies. The structure of the family in less developed societies has been of the extended kind, rather than the nuclear kind found in the industrialized world. This extended family means that the old are very much part of everyday family life and have an active role to play in the household. Where traditions and religious beliefs are important in a society, these, too, emphasize the importance of the old, with their acquired and accumulated wisdom. In industrialized societies, the uselessness of the old, the fact that they have little contribution to make, is emphasized by the paramount importance of the nuclear family. We live in a culture which values the new and has little interest in maintaining traditions passed on through the family—and this prejudice is reinforced by the accompanying failing health or impaired faculties of the aged.

There is also a contrast between West and East. Most of us know of the deep respect felt by the Chinese for their aged; this does not stem entirely from a tradition of ancestor worship, but also from a respect for knowledge acquired through experience.

This respect for the aged, though it exists, has been less obvious in the West.

Let us therefore take a look at a few communities—not belonging either to the East or West—for a more impartial view.

Among the most primitive people living today are those in the highlands of New Guinea. Here there are echoes of a primeval world, for these people have a pre-pottery, Stone Age culture. They go almost naked and live in grass huts. Inter-tribal wars are common, in which the males are often killed in large numbers. It puzzled me, when I was living among these people, what happened to their very old, for we often judge the cultural status of a people by the way they treat the dependent members of the community.

It was some time before I discovered the answer. One day I was passing between two villages on a mountain track when two girls, prettier than average, came and joined our little caravan. As we traveled along, they started to point out items of interest: "flame of the forest," the largest flower in the world, seen high in the trees from a distance; the New Guinea edition of the sloth; the cuscus; and some unusual birds.

Then, as we approached the next village, the girls beckoned to us in a very excited way until we stood at the threshold of a neatly made little hut with its own barred and well-used forecourt. Looking toward the entrance they started to call, indicating to us to have patience. Suddenly we heard movements from beyond the hut's dark entrance, as something white appeared amid the gloom, and soon we discerned a mop of white hair, and beneath it a very ancient face. Then the creature emerged into the daylight, unblinking in the strong sunlight, for she could not use her eyes. The girls kept calling the ancient woman. She followed the sound of their voices, coming slowly across to where we were standing. As she moved, her long white toenails made a clicking noise on the ground. Her fingernails had also grown long, but otherwise she was just skin and bone, her breasts flapping flatly against her skinny belly. She was not entirely naked, having on a wispy grass skirt. She came to us in a crouching position, croaking as she came. The girls indicated that we could go into the little compound, and though this was several years ago I can still feel the touch of those claws on my palm as I looked down on this face sans teeth, sans eyes, sans everything. But her mind was still lucid apparently, and the girls, it was plain to see, understood everything that she had to say. She held her hand in mine for about five minutes.

Suddenly, there was another noise from inside the hut, and out came a large and ancient pig. This, they said, was what kept the old lady warm in the chilly nights in West Irian. Food of the simplest variety was brought to her by the villagers. It is interesting, and instructive, that these people, one of the most "primitive" groups living, show much consideration for the very old.

However, in sharp contrast there is a very different custom to be found in other parts of West Irian. In some villages in this region they put the old person in a pit by the side of a busy track so that passers-by can throw in a stone, eventually burying the old person alive. These two extremes of treatment occur among people living only about 150 miles apart—although the people who practice these extremes probably never meet.

On the mainland of Southeast Asia, attitudes to the old also vary. In Thailand there is a large Chinese community. Among these people there is a tradition of care for the old that dates from time immemorial and is still firmly entrenched in mainland China itself. But take the average middle-class Thai family, the recent relatively rich; theirs is perhaps the most significant attitude, especially from a humanitarian point of view. The middle-class houses are placed in a compound with a moat or a wall, or even both, around it. In the center of the plot is the chief house where the nuclear family lives—father, mother and children. The material life of the household revolves around the kitchen on the ground floor; on the spiritual level it focuses on the chapel upstairs. During the day the kitchen is always the center of activity—here one will meet the seven ages of man on any normal evening. A gathering of twenty people, with ages ranging from one to ninety years, is commonplace. And, as if this is not large enough, adopted children or orphans may be brought into the family. An old lady of ninety sits teaching her great-granddaughter how to place her hand in one of the many classical dances. She is the

great-aunt of the household and lives in one of the little houses
that act as lodge gates. There are other small houses at the corners
of the compound where other elderly relatives live, ending their
days peacefully and securely.

Ninety years of age is very old for the Thai race; even sixty-five
is a good age. They would not dream of accepting that only two
people occupy a house; instead, all generations live together.
Under these circumstances, there is no need for old people's
homes. They regard our idea of putting all the old people together
under one roof as quite reprehensible. The old are much too valuable to the community; in their heads is most of the oral history,
the legends, folklore, the fairy tales for the children, the knowledge of the complicated dances, of their culture, the art of em-
broidery and points of general behavior. In modern society the
old also act as baby sitters. For this society, the separation of the
life of the old from the rest of the family is abhorrent and un-
desirable.

Many of these attitudes are dictated by racial origin, life-style
and environment. Most of these people lead a more active physical life than people in most Western countries; their bones, organs
and brains thus receive a more plentiful supply of blood, and they
do not atrophy so easily. This keeps them vigorous for a much
longer time. We in the West grow old gradually, whereas in many
Eastern countries people age very quickly at the end—suddenly
all bodily functions deteriorate in a year. This can cause some
surprises—I have met vigorous people who, a year later, have
become fragile old men.

Age, and attitudes to it, vary considerably. Age is influenced
by race, customs, diet and general attitudes to life. The communities that are the most age-conscious are often those that start
aging the earliest.

Up to now genetics have been thought of as the key to the mystery of aging. Unquestionably genes play a part in longevity (or
lack of it), and in isolated cases of individuals or families we have
searched for an explanation in the study of the aging cell. But environmental explanations should be carefully explored in the cases
where longevity (or early senility) is found in significantly large

numbers in whole communities where genetic connections do not always exist. Such a series of communities I investigated in Ecuador—communities unconnected often by racial factors, but having in common certain environmental factors. These last were those we explored.

2

Ecuador—Quito and
Vilcabamba

Before embarking on encounters with the centenarians of the
Andes, I will describe the history and terrain of the area in which
they live—an area full of interest and beauty.

Ecuador, on the west coast of South America, is wedged between Colombia to the north and Peru to the south and east. Until
recently it covered a much wider area, but Peru acquired her less
powerful neighbor's southern territory, the last confrontation
being in 1942.

Ecuador is naturally divided into three parts, the divisions
running from north to south. In the west lies the hot, tropical
coastal region; then comes the sierra, the region of the Andean
mountain chain, and the plateaus and valleys among these
mountains. Most of this region lies 1,525 meters above sea
level. Some of the Indians live up to a height of 4,300 meters, but
higher than that man cannot live. The scenery here is grand—high,
open and broken rolling hills, with the occasional snow-capped
mountain, such as Cotapaxi, looking very much like Japan's
Mount Fuji. This region is quite thickly populated, Mestizo (people of mixed Indian and Spanish blood) forming the bulk of the
population. Most of the larger cities of the sierra are on the plains,
except for Guayaquil, which is a seaport. The climate of the big

cities in the sierra is temperate. Where the centenarians so far have been found the climate is warmer, the altitude being between 1,375 meters and 1,525 meters above sea level, while that of the cities is between 2,450 and 3,350 meters. However, being close to the Equator (in fact the equatorial line passes just north of Quito) there is very little variety in the seasons. Some months have more rainfall than others, and there are plenty of fierce thunderstorms. But this is really the only seasonal variation.

The third region is the Oriente (or the eastern sector). Even today this has been little visited except by hunters, explorers and oilmen. It is an area of hot, steaming jungle, except where table-topped hills rise almost sheer out of it. It can be very unhealthy here—in more ways than one. It is an area with hostile Indians, who generally have the blow gun readily available. This region must have been more thickly populated at one time. Where some of the tree roots have grown out, often almost perfect ceramic specimens can be found of very unusual design; for example, two pots joined by an anthropomorphic figure.

The region in which Vilcabamba and the arc of centenarian villages are found, in the sierra, could be the cradle land of the South American people. There are signs everywhere of the effect of much human activity on nature—often too much for the present-day inhabitants of the high sierras to cope with. They have fled in their thousands from their native mountains, speeded on their way by the soil erosion of their own making; and their influx has often created problems in the cities of the region. In photographs taken of Quito around 1870 there were no Indians in sight among the population. Today, however, 75 per cent of the inhabitants are Indian.

The region of the Andes where the centenarians are found has been inhabited for many thousands of years. Remains of the earliest man found in the Americas, dating back thirty thousand years, come from Otovalo, a town quite close to the Ambuki district, where some very old people are found. From this early period onward, bones, artifacts (*obsidians*), pottery and earthworks indicate almost continuous occupation in the region. From pottery remains alone, there are indications of at least six cultures. All, though, existed before the Incas became more powerful than the other tribes in the Cuzco valley. They came north and conquered Quito forty years before the conquistadores came and took the city in 1534 (though the Spaniards had been in Ecuador since 1526).

Those who visit Ecuador today and see this evidence of man's activity, and who know little about the Americas, would be puzzled why, if the ancestors of the American Indian really came to that continent via the Bering Straits landbridge (which is thought by many to be the case), they did not stop off on their journey south at the highly desirable regions, such as California, and build up a civilization there. It immediately raises doubts as to whether they really came that way. If they came from the old world, as some suggest, why didn't they bring the wheel and the skill of writing with them? They could have equally well come into the sierra region of Ecuador via the numerous rivers, e.g. the Mira and the Santiago from the coast, as the nearest remains of bones and obsidians are not very far from these watersheds.

The region has many mysteries. There is evidence of ruined pyramids of vast size in this particular part of the Andes; farther south, only a hundred miles east of Vilcabamba, in Moruna province and the Cordillera Zaquarzongo, the mountains are honeycombed with beautifully made subterranean passages that cover a region seventy miles in one direction alone. Why were these made? There is also the mysterious double wall, twenty-five miles long. What was this to protect, and from whom?

The earthworks consist mainly of field systems, irrigation systems, ruins of villages, temples and towns, so ancient that they have become artificial mountains, rivaling the Middle Eastern "tells" or cities, built on the rubbish and remains of previous houses. All contain masses of potsherds. Even more fascinating are the *tollas,* or the tombs of the pre-Inca peoples, very similar to the round barrows of Salisbury Plain in England. If these tollas are excavated, more often than not they reveal many gold objects and superb pottery, usually of a polychrome variety, often beautifully glazed. Few of the local people bother to investigate them; their country is so full—to us—of the unusual. Archaeologically it is almost untouched—yet it has much to offer the archaeologist, as well as the historian and anthropologist.

Ecuador is not only rich archaeologically speaking, but is also richly endowed with natural resources. The country has been colonized since 1534, first by the Spaniards, and the development of these resources was to the benefit of the colonizers. Since 1819 there have been forty presidents, an indication that the country has not been stable, peaceful or conducive to development. On any mountain, mineral wealth, chiefly iron and copper, can be seen. There are in some places, easy of access, signs of old mining activities; those are quite obvious, but to what era to assign them is very difficult, and only where tools or potsherds are found is this possible. The rarer minerals are also found in many areas. Near Cuenca, quicksilver (mercury) oozes out of the rocks. Look in any of the numerous rivers and it will not be very long before you find gold dust in the sand, or tiny particles of gold. (I found looking for gold a very relaxing occupation!) The province of Esmeraldas in northeast Ecuador is so named after the great quantity of emeralds that are to be found there. At the sides of some of the rivers that flood there are many gold objects and artifacts, which the Indians often find and sell in the cities. These are often priceless, but, so that they will not be sent to museums, the Indians melt them down. The small gold objects found are modeled in the form of toads, alligators, insects and cats.

Much of the sierra has now been explored (though most of the Oriente is still waiting to reveal its secrets). Once I was traveling in the sierra, and we crossed one of the numerous small rivers, the deepest part only knee deep. However, soon afterward there was a terrific cloudburst that made it necessary to retrace our steps and, on our return to the ford, the whole river was a brilliant swirling yellow. We all looked up to the sun, but there was no sun; it was the gold particles in the water, stirred up from the river bottom, which had turned it yellow. The water, on our return, reached our waists.

The Spaniards could not penetrate all areas of the country and thus completely strip it of its riches, hardly surprising in a country of such high and broken terrain. There are some valleys of the sierra that are difficult even now to enter because of the constant landslides—Vilcabamba valley is one of these. The sierra has many natural beauties still remaining, chiefly of the type that cannot be destroyed, for the trees they can destroy, but the snow-capped mountains they cannot; of these, there are over a dozen including Cotapaxi and Cayambe.

For above all, Ecuador is a land of mountains, which increase the country's land surface and her transport problems. These mountains are all the more impressive for appearing so unexpectedly. For days the view will remain obscured; then, perhaps when the sun is fully up, the clouds shift, and there, like a city of the gods, is a magnificent snow peak, tinged pink in the morning sun. Ten minutes later, and again it is gone. Driving into Quito from the north in the early evening it is breathtaking to see the red sunset reflected on their white tips, the snow-capped guardians of the city. The conquistadores could not destroy all, but they saw to it that anything that it was possible to take back to Spain went there—to their churches and castles. They mined all the minerals they could, giving the Indians coca leaf to chew to make them more amenable to working the mines. All the Inca and pre-Colombian artifacts were melted down (most of these being profane) and thus, having destroyed these objects of cultural heritage, the Spaniards sent the gold and silver back in unartistic bars. How many of the beautiful Inca pectorals would go to make up one of these gold bars? They were so thin that you could almost blow them away, and they were of exquisite workmanship: many thousands must have been destroyed.

Where natural resources were concerned, the trees were probably the first to go, the Spaniards having no reafforestation program for their American colonies; these forests have never recovered, and the loss is great. Whenever they could the Spaniards felled the forests of the sierra, making huge *haciendas* (ranches) for themselves, and used the Indians here as they used them in the mines elsewhere—as cheap labor. Even until quite recently descendants of the Spanish invaders were allowed to mete out punishments that they thought fit on their Indian workers, having on the farms prisons—the wall fetters can still be seen. The teenage sons of the house were allowed to sleep with the Indian girls of the farm, and no woman on the farm was allowed to refuse the *don*.

Many of the Indians, not wanting to be so treated, fled to the higher sierras, and thus the denuding and overpopulation of the land went on for hundreds of years up and down the sierra, backed by the teaching of the Roman Catholic missionaries who followed the conquistadores to the Americas. The bubble burst in about 1880, when many Indians, unable to make a living in the sierras, came down in droves to Quito and the other cities. Fantasies and legends that cities and fortune were synonymous became more powerful. Their influx was aided by the roads and the railways that were built by the government, backed by cash from England—many a Victorian tycoon lost or gained his money in this way. Pictures and photographs of old Quito and towns built earlier show scenes remarkably similar to the Paris of the French Impressionists, although palm trees did not grow so vigorously in the squares of Paris as they do in the plazas of Quito.

The first Indian arrivals were caught in a familiar vicious circle. What little they had in their mountain homes they sold to get to the city to seek their fortunes. When they arrived there were no fortunes to be found, nor the means of returning whence they came. The tribal Indians still retain their dignified habits and customs, but the town Indians, in common with the Mestizos, seem first to ask of their surroundings, is this or that functional, what use can be made of it? If it is useful, they use it; if not, they destroy it. This extends to creatures as well as to material things; rarely does one see a boy without a catapult. At least one species of bird has found a way of avoiding the problem of becoming extinct—the parakeets, and some of the parrots, now fly very high and thus out of reach.

Many of the villagers are after the quick buck with a vengeance. It was found that the numerous terracotta figures that come to light when they are making soccer fields and new roads are popular with the tourists, so they have developed a factory for making them. Some of these fakes are very difficult to detect, the result being that many of the terracotta antiques of Ecuador are worthless today, for no one knows if they are genuine or not. Obviously the skill and techniques are still there, but put to rather negative ends. The Indian markets are also rather a disappointment. Essentially these markets deal in plastics, aluminum and tin —little, if anything, of their own culture is to be seen there. If a

piece of jewelry happens to sneak in, it commands a very high
price, often being bought by another Indian. The few wooden
items now made for sale bear the all too obvious marks of being
turned by machine. This rejection of the impressive aspects of
their own past and culture, and the preoccupation with Western
values, may account for the fact that the extraordinary centenarians have not been investigated until very recently. Their
own culture and achievements are considered of little value or interest.

In the cities there is the usual tension and conformity, the latter
seen in the overdressed Indians, the Mestizos in their thick serge
suits, and the horror of the people at seeing a visitor wearing
climbing boots, although mountains surround them. They will
often stand and gaze at such unseemliness, as people seeing someone caught naked would stare in our own society.

Unlike most of the South American capital cities, in Quito there
is a large part of the picturesque old Spanish colonial section still
standing. Most of the other countries on that continent, being
much richer than Ecuador, ruthlessly and efficiently replaced the
old with poor-quality new, in some places already crumbling.
(They are, however, now beginning to regret this, and Ecuador
has found that its relative poverty has been in this respect advan-
tageous.) The upper-class population used to live in the old town
but a few years ago they built new houses for themselves in one of
the suburbs and now rent out the old houses as apartments and
hotels.

I spent some time in Quito, and thus had an opportunity to observe city life at first hand. I wanted to explore the rumors I had
heard about the existence of the centenarians in southern Ecuador. I had already heard vague stories about a village called Vilcabamba where the inhabitants were supposed to live to a very
great age, but such stories occur in many regions and are nearly
always bogus, so, before going south, I wanted some confirmation.

I set out for an appointment in Quito with Dr. Acosta-Solis, for
I had been told he was an authority on southern Ecuador. I found
the house where he lived and worked, built in the traditional
Spanish style around a central courtyard. Passing through a cheap
paperback bookshop on the ground floor, I climbed the stairs, and

thinking I had reached the right place knocked on the partitioned door. It was ajar; confronting me was a sober soul carrying a chamber pot in one hand, an unlit candle in the other, and with a floppy nightcap on his head. I beat a hasty retreat and tried the next door.

This time I was more successful, and a sparkling bright-eyed girl of about eleven let me in and showed me into the book-lined room to await Dr. Acosta-Solis. Outside, the sun was shining, but not in that room; the shutters were only half open and the room was full of the stale, dank smell of old plants and papers.

The doctor confirmed that there was definitely some truth in the rumors of a village of centenarians, although beyond that he could not, or would not, commit himself. However, that was enough to make me determined to go south. He told me that the usual way that people reached the south and Loja—the capital of the southern province and the nearest town to Vilcabamba—was by air to Guayaquil, Ecuador's port and largest city. Then there was an army plane that would take one to the airstrip for Loja, although the airstrip and the town were separated by a distance of forty-five kilometers and a mountain range of 4,000 meters. "Or," he said, "one can go by bus." Then, looking at me very hard: "There is a bus that goes from Plaza de Commandant here in Quito some mornings and if you are lucky it will take you twenty-four hours, but it is best to stop the night at Cuenca." Then, as if talking to himself, he said: "Yes, that is the way for the naturalist—you see so much more of our country that way!"

He also suggested that I should contact Professor Orcez Villagomez, who had been collecting zoological specimens all over Ecuador; he would know where people who lived to be a great age were to be found.

I found Professor Orcez in his laboratory, in the department of political science, where I mentioned my quest to him. He gave me several leads; he also told me that his friend Dr. Miguel Salvador could tell me more. He was an internationally known heart specialist, living in Quito, and had just returned from Loja. He had been on the lookout for villages in which to study heart conditions, and he had come across one village where all the people seemed to be very ancient. Professor Orcez advised me to try to look him up as quickly as possible, as he was due to go to a conference.

During the next few days I met Dr. Miguel Salvador several times; he was a fund of information, and enthusiastic for me to go and visit the people. It seemed from what he said that they lived in a suburb of Loja (later the remote village was found to be forty-five kilometers away, along a road that on some days was not a road!). Many North Americans, especially doctors interested in genetics, had been asking him for information. No one, as far as I could make out, had entertained the idea that there were other factors than genetic ones at work.

I decided, as I had been advised by Dr. Acosta-Solis, to make the approach by road for then I could see the whole of the central part of Ecuador; Loja was about eight hundred kilometers from Quito and the road meandered through some of the most interesting parts of the Andes. The air flight entailed several long stops and would hardly let me see anything.

I had time for a further meeting with Dr. Salvador. He gave me more statistics on the people, this time on the cholesterol content of their blood, which was very low. Although Dr. Salvador's spoken English was not very fluent, he could read the language well and was widely read in European literature on cardiology. He is respected not only in Ecuador but among the international community of specialists in his subject. He also seemed to have a very prosperous practice. We discussed the people of the valley and the findings of his survey and he said that he would very much like to see any report that I might make on the people. I showed him the composite interview forms which we had devised to obtain information on diet and health that I had brought from the universities of Birmingham and London, and what I proposed to do—to carry out a survey on their teeth, physique, diet and the occurrence of all the diseases they had had.

He himself seemed convinced that everything connected with these people living to a very old age and having strong hearts had a genetic cause; that they were members of old Spanish families who had settled in the little town after the battle of Pichincha in 1827, and that all the old people were members of a certain few families that had inter-married; and that their longevity was helped along by a low calorie diet. He gave me copies of all the relevant statistics in his possession. Where heart disease was concerned, he said, they were extraordinary. Out of the 338 he had managed to examine in Vilcabamba only one person showed signs of having a weak heart. He added that his friend Dr. Jorge Santiana, a cancer specialist, had also visited the place and that he had only found one growth, benign, on a very elderly person. The town had, in fact, the lowest incidence of these diseases that he had ever heard of. It was also true that the people there were often of great age.

These two doctors, however, being specialists, had concentrated on the branch of study that had interested them. Yet both, in their specialist fields, had found the Vilcabambans to be remarkable people and hoped to go and visit them again. They considered them to be remarkable specimens of humanity, but could not see the interest that they would have beyond their own field.

I still had a few days to spare so I visited some other people who knew what was of interest in their country. I was told of two places where I could find centenarians. One was called Manta on the coast. An article written a few years ago entitled *A Man from Manta* was shown to me: this man was reputed to be 127 years old. The other centenarian was a man of 125, again living on the coast of Ecuador.

However, they had missed the point, I felt, for they were telling me of isolated individuals; this could simply mean that one person had particular stamina and was remarkable as an individual. It is when there is a large number of centenarians in one area that the place and *environment* become significant—a very important difference. In such cases it becomes important to study the possible effects of the environment on health and the aging process.

I felt, from these anecdotes, that the first group to study was the one near Loja. I thought it was definitely worth trying to see if their diet, or something else in their environment, was the cause of their longevity and good health. Certainly I felt their environment might hold the key, and I began to look further into it, with a great sense of excitement. For if there was an area where communities of people lived not only to a great age, but to a healthy, lucid and agile old age, would it not be interesting to discover whether there were things to be learned for our own society?

I looked at Loja on the map and saw that it was surrounded by mountains of about the same height as the places where the other, unauthenticated, centenarians had been found—in the Caucasus (the Abkhasians) and in Pakistan (the Hunzas). I noticed that the majority of the isolated individual centenarians to be found in Ecuador lived close to the sea and had been fishermen. (In my previous dietary surveys of living "primitive" peoples I often found individuals living to a great age near the coast.) However, those in the other two regions of the world were small holders like the people near Loja. Someone mentioned the name of Vilcabamba but only in passing, and as I could not see it marked on any map I put it down as a suburb of Loja.

After a conversation with a man from the government some months earlier I had been encouraged to embark on this trip. I wondered if this was still possible as there had been a coup d'état since then. However, the government seemed just as delighted as previously to hear that I was going, although special permission had to be obtained as the region was in a sensitive border area. They gave me the names of people whom I should contact when I was there, such as Dr. Gonzales, the Chief of the Public Health. I also visited the World Health Organization (WHO) representative and he advised me to approach this same man when I arrived at Loja.

One of the boys at the hotel where I was staying, Victor Sánchez, noticed my preparations for the south. He came to see me one evening, and told me that he was born in Vilcabamba, that it was in fact a long way from Loja, and very difficult to get to. Also that there *were* some ancient people living there, in fact a considerable number of them. He came from a very large family, and thus had had to leave to earn a living, though he had been very unhappy to do so. His description of the area made it sound even more interesting and I had no hesitation whatever in deciding that this was the place to visit, however difficult it might be to reach.

3

Loja, and the Search for the Centenarians

A long-distance bus journey is probably one of the best ways of seeing a country and getting to know about its people. The journey from Quito to Loja was certainly no disappointment in this respect. As there was no form of lavatory on the bus, and the first stop was not for some hours, my fellow travelers were using the wall or the back of the bus to ensure comfort on the journey. The bus, a powerful Mercedes, had remarkably good tires but, although the roads required tires of the best, bald and worn tires were more common than not. All luggage—great blanket-covered bundles, piles of skins, livestock and dead animals—was thrown on the rack on the top of the bus.

There were not many passengers: a couple of youths sitting near me, the usual group of Indians taking their usual places at the rear of the bus, some women with mysterious baskets and voluminous shawls, as well as a sprinkling of potential high-jacking guerrilla types with bottles of drink in their hip pockets.

Just before the bus pulled into the first police post on the southern highway for the routine police search, the conductor produced from nowhere a smart cap with a badge. This cap sat on the top of his mass of black curly hair. As soon as we had pulled away, after the police survey of the poultry (which was the bulk of what was on the roof), the cap was chucked to one side, the community sank into informality and the bottles of drink came out.

The two youths near me, who were not drinking, produced apparently from thin air a sedate little pink phonograph, and started to play those cheap records that I have not seen outside Ecuador. One of the tunes was a haunting melody called "Carnival de la Vida." Fragments of this song kept coming through the roar of the engine, the grinding of the gears and the blaring of the bus radio, but, as we climbed up toward the snow line, the power of the radio seemed to diminish considerably, and "Carnival de la Vida" won the contest.

The bus traveled on through wild country, with mountains soaring up from the flat plains, the local inhabitants struggling across apparently trackless landscape, carrying loads of potatoes and peat, with mountain mists swirling all around.

After four hours and a gradual descent of many thousands of feet, we arrived at Riobamba. Instantly the bus was besieged by hordes of people, of all sizes and ages, selling a kind of pressed dried fruit for which the town is famous. The driver abandoned the bus and the street sellers tried to get on as the people tried to get off—a general mass of squeezing and shoving humanity. This is the usual result of any stop, and if the stop is a short one the pushing and shoving continues until the driver appears with the conductor, yelling out the bus's destination—in this case shouting "Cuenca, Loja." If the passengers have not managed to get on the bus before it starts, that is just too bad. Some of the vendors may even get carried along the way, and unless they are very persuasive they do not get put off before the bus reaches its next stopping point—often many hours later.

After crossing a high desert-like region and climbing yet another mountain range, where the clouds hung far below, the bus reached Cuenca just before darkness fell. The town seemed oppressive, with drunks lying on the streets and church bells tolling, seemingly everywhere. I had intended to stop the night there and to catch a bus at some very early hour the next morning. But when I returned to the bus station I found the bus almost ready to depart though it had only stopped there for a little over an hour.

The driver, who had already been at the wheel for over seventeen hours was tense but ready to continue.

Most of the faces were new, but the two young men were still sitting nearby, one clutching the pink phonograph and the other the handle, ready to start up and entertain the bus once more with that haunting little melody.

So we started off into the night. Then the rain started, heavy rain that beat against the window. There were no lights anywhere and as we began to climb it began to get colder. The road seemed no more than a mud track, and the bus just slid around the bends. After nearly four hours we reached the halfway point, and through the pouring rain we could see neat coffee tables in a long low room with a storm lantern swinging from the rafters. The entire load of passengers ran through the rain to this haven—pink phonograph and all. Soon we heard another bus pull up. It had come from the opposite direction—from Loja, our own destination. The sodden driver with two passengers came through the rain. The driver made straight for the driver of our own bus, and under the now popping storm lantern they spoke in low voices, occasionally breaking off to stare into the stormy night.

The brief respite was soon over and back to the bus and to "Carnival de la Vida" we went. The rain came down in sheets over the first mountain range for two thousand miles of the Amazon basin. The two young men with the phonograph started dozing, as were the rest of the passengers; the driver just stared ahead. His numerous cigarettes were lit and shared by his codriver. We were all close to sleep.

Suddenly we were conscious that the bus was not moving any more, and there before us was a moving mountain of slurry. There was no road ahead, but a mass of ooze, seemingly coming out of the side of the mountain. I was waiting for the shovels and torches to come out, but the driver backed up the road. He was backing without a light; they had no refinements like reversing lights, or even torches, so I lent them mine. The engine was revved fiercely and then it charged forward at the moving slurry until it could move no farther into the mass. We were now surrounded on all sides by the slurry which slowly but determinedly started to drag the bus toward the edge. Soon the bus had quite a tilt and things were starting to fall from the luggage racks. But the lights of a lorry were seen through the rain coming from the other side. Its driver, deciding that discretion was the better part of valor, stopped at the edge of the slurry. The two young men hastily fled to the bus's exit, letting the phonograph fall to the floor. As they passed me they said, "We no like, we frightened." Only when I saw the lights of a town far down in the valley beneath did I realize the reason for their haste; we were hanging on the edge of a precipice. Most of the others seemed too tired or too drunk to bother moving.

The bus seemed to start a slow waltz, and was already partly over the edge when a rope was thrown from the lorry and tied to the front of the bus, and with the engine of our bus working at full throttle we were saved from the abyss.

Just along the road there was a shrine dedicated to St. Christopher and here all the passengers, now thoroughly awake, got out to pay their respects to the patron saint of travelers, who has to work hard on these Andean roads. "Carnival de la Vida" started up once more, the phonograph obviously none the worse for its tumble, and our journey continued.

We soon saw the lights of Saraguro and the Indian settlement, and not long afterward the electric lights of Loja far down in the valley. Then, an hour or two before dawn, the bus rolled into one of the plazas of the town.

To arrive in Loja town as one usually does, at about four o'clock in the morning, and see figures grouped around a cross as they forge forward through the driving rain, singing a dirge as they go, is eery. These religious ceremonies are not uncommon, but they give a strange effect, especially at this time of morning; there is generally a priest there in his robes. This sight, and the battered bus that had crossed the mountains, spattered with mud and slurry, and the driver and the passengers with two days' growth of beard, made me think about travel in the old coaching days.

The city of Loja lies on the floor of a long valley; two rivers, the Malacatos and the Zamora, run more or less parallel for most of its length, and the houses and streets are built along these. The streets are straight, and there are five plazas—in some cases with very old houses around them. One plaza at the northern end of the town has an ancient colonial church dating back to 1535. Most of the original town has been destroyed by the numerous earthquakes it has suffered. During the few days that I spent there on my way to Vilcabamba, the inhabitants often told me how there had been tremors—usually at night or in the early morning.

At first sight it seemed rather a drab town, with its colorless houses, its straight streets, and its regiments of shops and dull cafes. But some of the plazas, with their pretty shrubs, trees and flowers, can look attractive; and there are the occasional old houses. Some of these have beautiful doors, made of one massive piece of wood with mysterious door handles of brass. One such shows a hand complete with the frilled sleeve; the thumb, which is folded over, and the under sleeve, show in exquisite detail the nail and the lace. These houses have superb balconies of cast iron. There are no glazed windows—only shutters, similar to those of the houses in the older towns of Thailand.

Some of these houses, too, could tell a tale, for they were already built when the conquistadores marched through with their Inca prisoners. In the old opulent palaces, the gigantic beams and panels tell of huge forests in the area. What a contrast with the environs of Loja now! Very few trees are allowed to grow, though some enterprising people have recently attempted to make avenues along some of the roads.

Late in the evenings, when the hustle and bustle which the Indians bring to the town is over, the town seems full of gurgling sounds from the small rivers rushing through it. The Lojans love these rivers, for they sometimes still bring gold along—right into the town. The women find it when they are washing clothes, using the larger stones as scrubbing boards. This adds much more enthusiasm to washing day! Usually the clothes are carried down in enormous wooden trenchers that in Europe would have pride of place at any banquet—a further indication of the natural wealth that was once found in this place.

But this is not the only contribution that the rivers have to offer to the Lojans. The main river, always referred to as "the Golden River," has inexhaustible supplies of stone that can be taken from it for building purposes. No matter how many they take out of it, there always seems to be more, and neither of the rivers has ever been known to dry up. Even though they are proud of the rivers, the Lojans abuse them by throwing in most of their rubbish; in this way it acts as a sewer.

No matter what hour of the day or night one promenades along the river banks, a strange and plaintive cry will be heard, very difficult to locate. Whatever creature makes the noise is a master of ventriloquism. Does it come from the small trees that grow beside the river, or from the bundles of lush grass that also grow there?

The smaller river, the Zamora, after it leaves Loja valley meanders slowly through many beautiful canyons and gorges. The only route between Loja and Zamora (the main center of population in the Oriente) follows the river's course. The Loja valley was one of the first to be colonized by the Spaniards, in the year 1535, probably because of its associations with Atahualpa, who sometimes took refuge in the Palmyra valley (just beyond Vilcabamba) in times of trouble.

The town has many moods; the worst is in the rain, when it becomes covered with mud. The groups of Indians do much to liven it up. They seem more numerous on some days than others. They are the Saraguro Indians—wearing striking homespun clothes with wide, thick, pale-colored hats (some weighing up to twelve pounds); mostly they gather near the market and around the central plaza—they have been doing the same for centuries. Their numbers are dwindling—at most there are eight thousand of them, but they are so conspicuous that they seem more numerous.

There is a remarkable contrast between the sexes. The women have little round faces that go well with their broad hats, and the men have long thin faces, with great craggy noses and deep-set dark eyes. They believe that they are the direct descendants of the Incas. There is certainly nothing cringing or servile about them, even when they have been drinking—which is very often. They occupy the nearby small towns of Saraguro and San Lucas, but they may turn up anywhere—sometimes on the hills above Vilcabamba. These tall, gaunt men have odd habits and mannerisms that are very engaging. Their faces seem full of character when compared with those of the button-nosed Indians of the rest of Ecuador.

The apparent drabness and dullness of the valley make the

surprises more dramatic when they come. For instance, I have never seen anywhere else in South America the variety of hummingbirds that frequent the gardens. These are almost impossible to shoot or bring down with a catapult and even the larger ones thrive there. The birds add much to the gaiety of the region.

Loja was also the first place where I tasted the cedron drink, made from the leaves of the tree; either fresh or dried leaves are used, and hot water is poured onto them. The bushes grow in the gardens and hedges, and anyone who grew it commercially for export would be a wealthy man.

The large central market is another center of attraction. Here all the vessels used to display the food and the flowers are wooden trenchers. Many Indians and country people are to be seen there selling their wares. Some of these are very attractive—flowers, such as the arum lily—and some repulsive, like entrails and raw pigskin.

The average Lojan is extremely conservative. Fathers still read any letters received by their daughters; if a girl is known to have lovers, then her marriage prospects are nil. If a husband on the wedding night believes his wife not to be a virgin he feels highly insulted, renounces her and sends her back to her parents. They pride themselves on being very Spanish; in fact they excel in bad Spanish customs at the expense of the good ones. Hospitality rarely extends beyond the coffee cup, whoever the host or the guest. However, when a meal is offered it is all the more appreciated.

On my arrival in Loja I detected a range of long buildings made of adobe with large barred windows. At first I thought that, at best, it was some form of a railway station, at worst, a prison or an asylum; but I discovered that there was no railroad to Loja, and that it was the hospital. This is very primitive, to say the least. Some of the beds are in the basement, and the street dirt enters through the unglazed windows. Lack of a large enough budget accounts for the state of the hospital; now they hope to build a new one, and plans are already underway.

Before I came to Loja I was given to understand that it was in Loja that the old people lived. It was only through a considerable amount of questioning of doctors in Loja that I discovered that

Vilcabamba was the place they had meant. Victor Sánchez had been right. In fact, there *are* many old people to be seen in Loja on market days, in ponchos and other dress of the country people; they come several miles into town, and look exactly like the country people on the small holdings that are around Vilcabamba. It would be interesting to study these people and the districts they come from in the future; this time we could not because of the large geographical distance between these people and the Vilcabambans.

To study the people of Vilcabamba, it was necessary to spend time in Loja to look at the many records, and to talk to people who could offer some information about them. Dr. Hugo Gonzales was able to give me statistics of individual centenarians, their health and the treatment that they had been receiving. There was quite a lot of information on their health, e.g. the state of their lungs, heart, liver and whether they suffered from rheumatism. Medical treatment often entailed giving out unnecessary pills, sometimes locally made, of no medicinal value, which did more harm than good. Penicillin and cortisone were sometimes used indiscriminately. Appendectomy before proper investigation, hepatic abscesses which can be left, were among operations I discovered had been performed. But I do not believe the very ancient people still living on their farmsteads in the mountains have been much affected by the pills and operations. It is only very recently that doctors, or anyone else, have been able to get through to Vilcabamba and the other villages we later found, as what track there was, was being constantly washed away; recently (December 1973) they have made a road through.

To the people of Loja, who were Catholics, Vilcabamba with its healthy centenarians was seen as a place of miracles. But at Quito they took a more practical view of the matter, simply saying that "there are some very interesting specimens of humanity at Vilcabamba."

My next step was to find out how to reach the fabled village. I had been lucky in the extent of help I received from the government authorities, but I felt that I should like to get there first of all incognito, just in case it was a government show place.

On inquiry at some of the market shops, I found that a kind of cattle truck went to Vilcabamba about once a week, at around 11 A.M., and there were some seats in it for passengers. I soon found the agency in a back street, and for twelve sucres I received a hand-written ticket for a seat on the vehicle, at 11 A.M. the next day.

Next morning I arrived at the bus station at 10 A.M., to find the section of the bus for cattle, behind the benches, completely full with pigs, chickens and a couple of bullocks. The benches, too, seemed packed. I took my seat, and for two hours had the ordeal of people and packets passing backward and forward, and people wanting to see to their animals. Then the bus was ready to depart. One of the bullocks, my nearest companion, started to snuffle in my pockets through the loose barrier between the human and animal sections.

The track to Vilcabamba lay for the most part along the sides of the mountain. Sometimes we descended to the floor of the valley to cross the river that lay there like a silver snake. To get over to the other side there was a rough-hewn bridge, with a canopy over it, as with all the bridges in that area, though what purpose this served I could never discover. We passed several villages, all with a fine population of babies, fighting cocks and curly-haired, sway-backed pigs.

Along the whole length of the ravine that we traveled for most of the thirty-five or so miles to Vilcabamba, there was much evidence of old Inca tracks and ways, and here and there the ruins of some ancient building, with its crumbling field walls. Several times the passengers had to leave the bus to remake the road, which had either slipped or been washed away during the previous night, for there was more or less perpetual rain. After this there was always a "Tally Hoo" on the horn to bring back those passengers who were busy "seeing to the back tire." Other stops were to allow cattle to cross, baby donkeys to seek their mothers, and for Muscovy ducks, which stood in front of the bus and hissed.

We soon arrived at a village called Vilcabamba. The girl beside me said, "It won't be long now." Over the next rise we saw a valley below us; the whole bus gave a sigh, and a universal cry went up—"Vilcabamba"—and there below us *was* Vilcabamba. In the center of the broad valley lay a large village and above the village, something like a halo! It was certainly the first large piece of blue sky I'd seen since arriving in Loja.

We descended to the valley floor, across a final rickety bridge, and ahead of us lay the streets of Vilcabamba. The houses were single story and of a ranch-house style. Down the street came a figure on horseback, complete with dog; it could have been a scene straight from a Western. Several of the passengers got out at this juncture, but I stayed to see how far we would go. The main stopping place proved to be the plaza. The bullock who had been trying his best to chew up my coat seemed really sorry to see me leave. It was lovely to get out into the late afternoon sunshine and feel the gentle cooling breezes from the mountain. Gold seemed to be the keynote of the scene. The square was dominated by a golden-colored church, and the whole of the plaza was a blaze of marigolds, and they in turn reflected the gleaming sunshine.

I made my way to the little cafe on the corner, where a rough kind of whiskey and some slabs of cheese were brought out. There were many wiry-looking women about with large daisy-covered hats and bare feet, but, as yet, no remarkable methuselahs. These I was to find later.

While gazing on the pleasant little plaza and the view all around, I could not help noticing a small mountain that rose up from the last of the gardens of the village. In fact it looked an ideal vantage point from which to survey the area and to take photographs of a panorama of the village. Perched on the top of this was a perfect little ranch house complete with verandah.

I made my way up the broad streets, past the grazing donkeys and Indian ponies and the friendly little dogs and long, wavy-haired pigs. All the people I met in the fifteen minutes I spent on that journey were most polite in their greetings. The road then became just a path, narrowed, meandered and steepened. I now met little children, also extremely friendly, and not at all afraid. I reached the verandah, and the site was perfect. In a few moments I was approached by several lean dogs, who romped and turned over on their backs around me.

The noise must have disturbed the owner, for soon a strong, pleasant-looking woman dressed in black emerged. With her was a servant, bare of foot but wearing the most charming of straw hats, all decked with flowers. (It was in fact a typical Sunday-school hat.) Her dress was rather faded, flowered, with a ragged hem. In Spanish and by indications they showed that they would be delighted if I took photographs from the verandah, and started to creep about on tiptoe, as if they would otherwise disturb the pictures. They began to clear an old table covered with books and storm lanterns, for the preparation of a meal.

4
The Environment of Vilcabamba

The valley of Vilcabamba has many peculiarities. It is interesting to speculate on whether the early inhabitants of the valley found its mysteries even more inexplicable than do its present ones. Certainly it has many extraordinary qualities—the plant life, the climate, the range of trees and crops growing there, its minerals, its dramatic mountains, and the remarkable regular 19° Centigrade midday temperature, which seems to stay more or less steady at all times of year. There is also a cooling wind that comes down from the mountains every day from 12:00 to 3:00 P.M. Above all, it has an extraordinary atmosphere, which is hard to put down to any single factor. The rainfall for the months is as follows (in millimeters):

January	81.7
February	105.7
March	92.9
April	49.5
May	50.0
June	18.9
July	1.0
August	3.2

September	15.3
October	87.6
November	123.9
December	49.2

which adds up to 678.9 mm.

Even the name of the village is intriguing. It has been suggested that the name means "Sacred Valley," derived from the language of the Quechua Indians: "Vilca"—sacred, and "Bamba" —valley. There is another possible root for its name. An interesting tree, much written about, grows (though less and less these days) in the vicinity of Vilcabamba. There are many indications— stumps, etc.—to show that it was more prolific there in the past. This is the Vilco or Wilco tree. Some say (mainly those of Spanish origin) that the valley gets its name from this tree. Plenty are found higher up the slopes of Mandango and Warango, the mountains that overlook Vilcabamba. There seems to be no reason why Vilcabamba should be picked out for its special home, especially since Indian names were at one time much more common. This tree is found—under such names as Tamarindo, Yoke and Yacoana —all over the central and northern part of South America, so the latter explanation does not seem particularly likely.

The tree is interesting. It is very attractive with fernlike leaves, decorative branches and pretty red fruit. It has many uses among which is the extraction from it of a hallucinatory drug. The Incas also made a snuff from it.

The canton of Loja is split up into urban and rural parishes. Vilcabamba is situated forty-five kilometers southwest of the town of Loja. A quarter of the canton's area belongs to Vilcabamba village itself and the rest belongs to the rural hamlets in the mostly mountainous country around. It is these hamlets which are the most interesting from a gerontological as well as a historical point of view. This region, at the time of the colonial wars in the early nineteenth century, gave shelter to many Spanish people.

Vilcabamba is placed at 79° longitude (west) and 4° 15′ 40″ latitude south, and it is between 1,520 meters and 1,700 meters above sea level. The rural population of the environs of the village is 3,555 and that of the village itself is 819. In area it is about 100 square kilometers. It is bounded on the north by the town of

Malacatos. Its natural division though is the cordillera east and
west, which unites at the little hamlet of Cerarengo, north of Vilcabamba. On the south it is bordered with Yangana and on the
west with the Cordillera Taranza, and in the east with the Eastern
Andean Cordillera.

The towering peak of Mandango (meaning the devil in the
Quechua language), 2,000 meters above Vilcabamba, looks at a
distance like some cathedral carved by nature out of the rock—or
a Noah's Ark stuck on Mount Ararat. But when one climbs up to
its base, a climb of several hours, one finds that the impression of a
pillared wall that one had from the valley floor is only an illusion;
for it is made up of water-worn pebbles and boulders, intermixed
with a natural mortar. The mixture would be far more at home on
the banks or the floor of some mighty and ancient river than up
there. How did the debris get up to those heights?

To the north of the village we find the ridge of Cararango, from
which there is a splendid view of Vilcabamba, with its houses
scattered all over the wide valley on the approach from Loja.
There is another ridge to the south, which is a place of many
legends and traditions relating to Inca times; it is close to Quinara.
Through this place passes the road to Yangana. In the region of
La Guaranga a great many varieties of excellent maize of different
colors are grown.

Surcumina is a steep-sided valley that looks as if a meteorite has
seared its way through the surface of the soil. This place is noted
for discoveries of gold in the past and occasionally it is found even
now, when the flood water comes. There is an Inca cemetery
there, too, not far from some strange pillars of rock that the elements have shaped grotesquely; it looks like nature's attempt to
form a Greek temple in the rock. There are also some very pleasant springs in the vicinity.

The Chamba, a warm river, is born out of the union of two
streams, the Yambala and the Capamaco; these at one time
formed the boundaries of some large haciendas between Loja and
Vilcabamba. The Uchima, in the eastern cordillera, flows through
the valley floor of Palmyra, and also receives here the icy melted
snow water from the ravines of Cachaco and Masanamaca. Gold
is found here too. Later it goes on to join the Catamayo (Pis-

cobamba). These two rivers, Chamba and Uchima, join near Vilcabamba.

There are many lakes in the hollows up in the mountains, but these cannot be seen from Vilcabamba itself. This is true also of San Pedro de la Bendita. Many of these lakes get their water supply from the mountain river of Masanamaca, which itself springs from a lake. A few of these lakes are now being used as reservoirs for the villages, and the supply of piped water comes from them. After heavy rain in the mountains, the flow of water can be an obstacle for travelers going to Yangana, for the bed of the river has to be crossed, and this can be a raging torrent or a trickle, depending upon the amount of overflow from these lakes. As the Chamba, Solander and the Malacatos flow into this river it becomes the great Catamayo, which winds its way over the border and into Peru.

There are several dried-up river beds, but these, after heavy falls of rain, can become very dangerous, as they become the channels for flash floods. One of these is the Iscaidido that, at such times, brings down quantities of gold from the towering heights of Lambonuma; it only has water running through it in the "winter." It also brings down with its flood a large quantity of valuable silt that is put on the crops. The silt arrives mixed with a black volcanic ash, quite a lot of which also passes into the river Chamba. The dried-up water courses make it very dangerous to cross rivers that flow across the roads, especially to Palmyra and Yangana.

To the east of Yamburara, and five hours by pack mule from the road, there is a marvelous area of ground called *pajonal* with masses of vegetation and grasses of many colors. Contrasting with this verdant pasture are fourteen lakes, all with very clear water. But people rarely go there—they prefer to stay in the inhabited regions. They say that this place is full of strange noises, but to me it appeared only to be the wind.

The largest of these lakes is called Margarita, from which runs the river Masanamaca. It is believed that the sand that forms a large part of the subsoil, at least in the Vilcabamba valley, was caused by many big rivers and glaciers bringing deposits into the plain, where the village now stands. This was at one time a lake bottom. The course of the rivers can be seen in the hanging valleys that have been carved out to form the five arms of a star, Vilcabamba occupying the center. They brought in great quantities of sand, gravel and silt, and with it calcium which is found also as a deposit, mingled to create this very fertile region. The surface of the land looks very similar to that of Loja. There occurred, at the end of Tertiary times, a raising of the land due to tectonic movement, and the lake disappeared; but the sub-geology remained more or less the same, with its wealth of mineral deposits.

Climbing up above the hacienda belonging to the "lady" of the village, Señora Río Frío, about two miles distant, one reached a region that had a peculiar pinkish soil. Here bubbled up the first of the small sacred springs where the village obtained its water at one time, and on certain days the people of the village make a pilgrimage for water there, although it has been much muddied by the feet of cattle. Farther up toward the ridge of Warango, about another two miles on, is yet another spring. This is supposed to be the most sacred spring of all, and remains untouched by cattle. As a result, when I scraped away the dead leaves it lay in a little flower-strewn dell, with water that was crystal clear. There were indications that the people had visited it for centuries, by the marks and signs on the surrounding rocks. Sixty meters above this was the top of the mountain that formed a kind of ridgeback. There were signs of agricultural activities all around that must have dated from Inca times. If one looked down toward where Vilcabamba lay, far down in the valley floor, a hill could be seen that obstructed most of the village from view, and where the woods did not hide the view there were many signs of early habitation. Stone hut circles could be seen, possibly Inca or even pre-Inca. If we turned to the other side there was a most interesting view—the tips of some mines showing yellowish white in the background, the river Piscobamba meandering in the foreground. A strong sense of the mystery and beauty of this historic area is engendered here.

The principal crops grown in this area are wheat and barley (on the mountain slopes), potatoes, yucca (a root) and maize. Grapes are also grown in small quantities—but in nothing like the quantities that could be grown. There are small valleys, such as Kinara, off the main one, where crops grow superbly. According

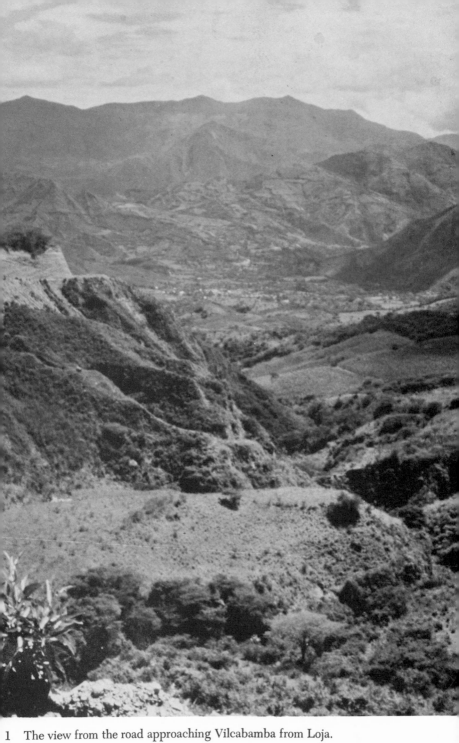

1   The view from the road approaching Vilcabamba from Loja.

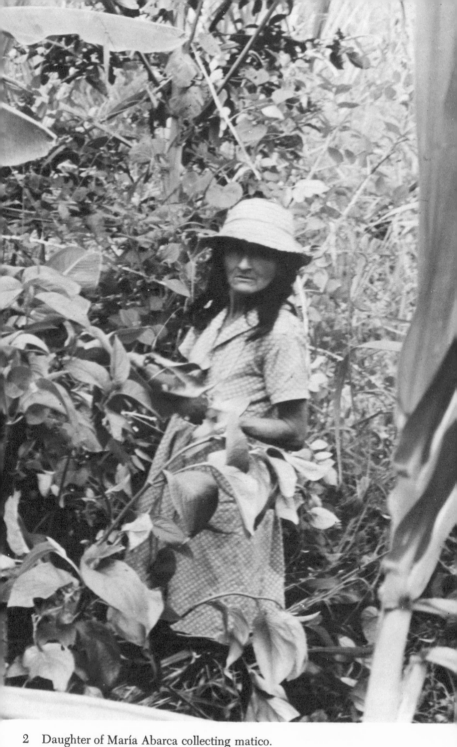

2 Daughter of María Abarca collecting matico.

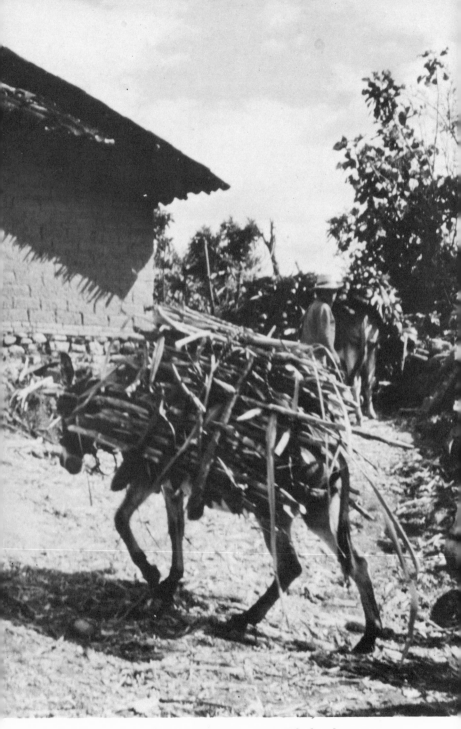

Bringing in the sugar cane for processing into rum in Vilcabamba.

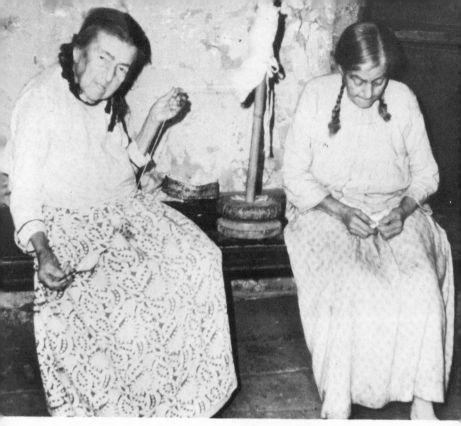

4 Two sisters, Pastora and Rosario Arias, spinning in San Pedro.

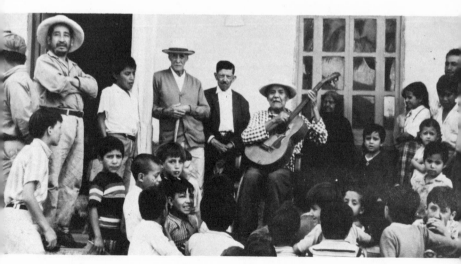

5 Samuel Rochas, aged 142 years, surrounded by children in San Pedro.

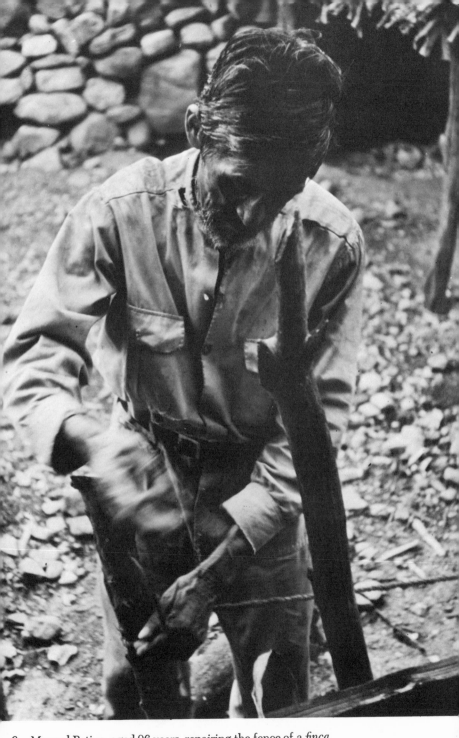

6   Manuel Patino, aged 96 years, repairing the fence of a *finca*.

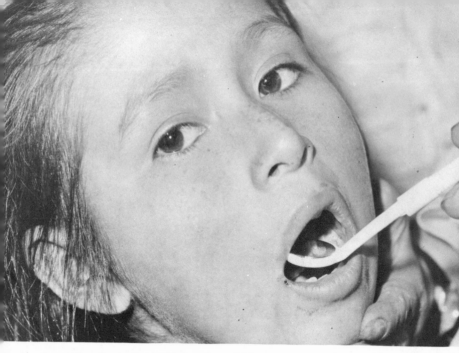

7   Inspecting the teeth of Vilcabamban children.

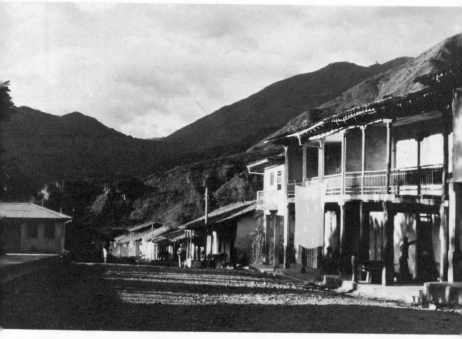

8   Village street, Vilcabamba.

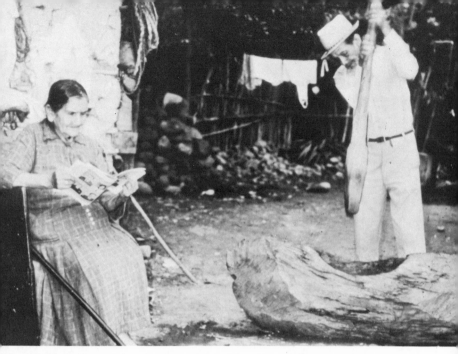

9 Clodovea Herrera, aged 110, reading without spectacles.

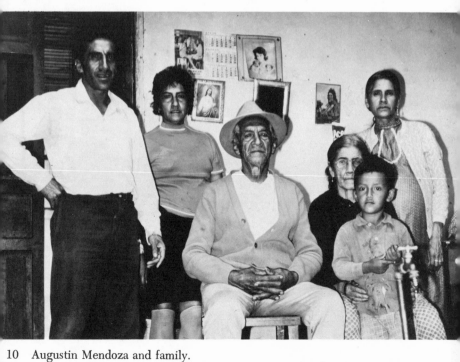

10 Augustin Mendoza and family.

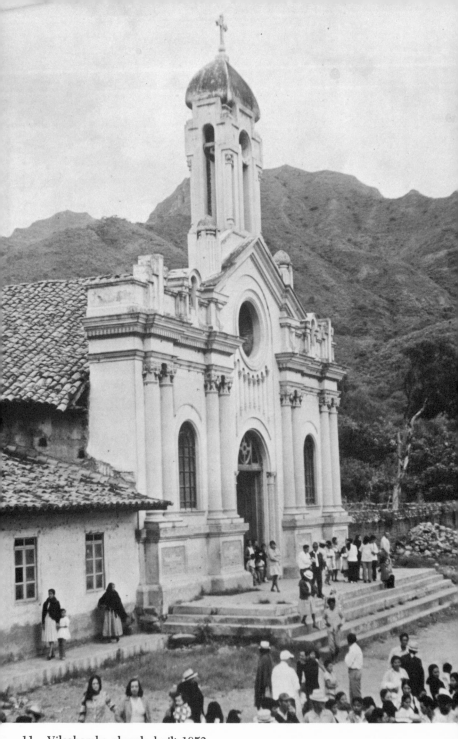

11 Vilcabamba church, built 1852.

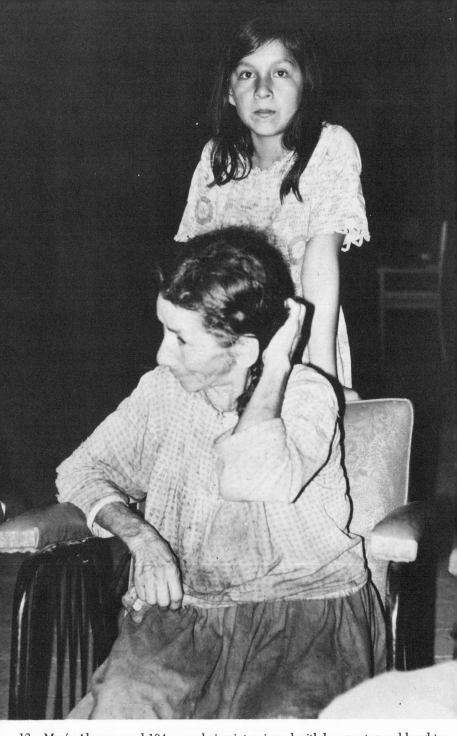

12 María Abarca, aged 104 years, being interviewed with her great-granddaughter, aged 11 years.

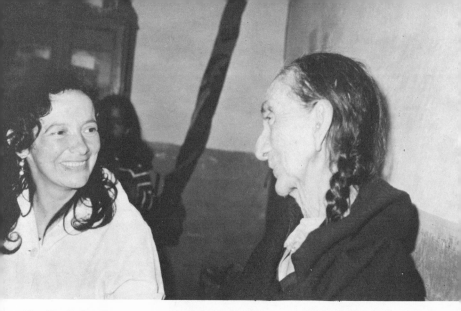

13   Dr. Lolita Samaniego with Dolores Mendieta, aged 97 years.

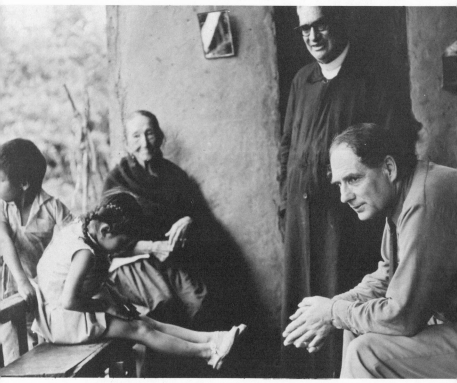

14   The author with Francisco Bravo (the priest of Vilcabamba) and Michael Mendieta Quesada, aged 106 years.

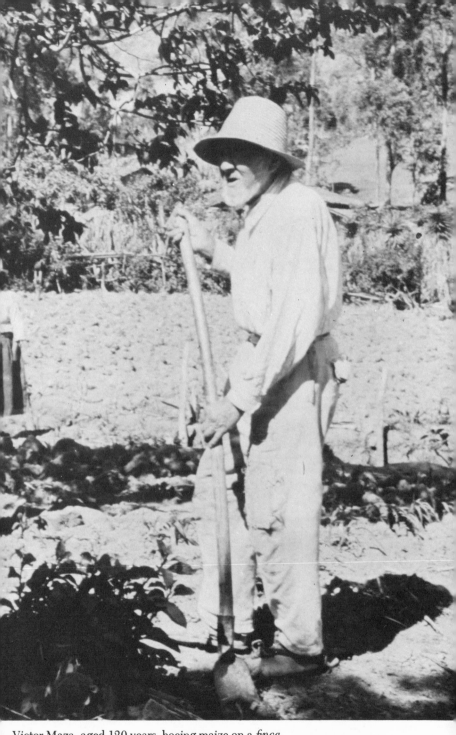

Victor Maza, aged 120 years, hoeing maize on a *finca*.

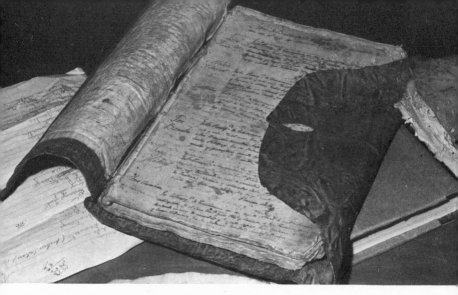

16 One of the books from which records of the ages of the centenarians were taken.

PARTIDA DE DEFUNCIONES

N. 235
Torres
José
María
(Adulto)

En la parroquia de *San Pedro de la Bendita*, diócesis de Loja, a *los vinticinco* días del mes de *Diciembre* del año del Señor de mil novecientos *treinta y tres* Yo *Carlos Alfonso Erreis, Cura* Párroco de la misma iglesia mandé dar sepultura eclesiástica al cadaver de *José María Torres* de edad de *ciento cincuenta* _____ feligrés de *esta parroquia*, vecino de *Molashe* hijo de *Eribio Torres y Saturnina Tinasco* fallecido en la Comunión de la Santa Iglesia el *día vinticinco del mes en curso* Se confesó con *el Dr. Dn. Juvenal Jaramillo*, recibió el Sagrado Viático el día _____ y la Extrema Unción el _____ Fué enterrado en *el cementerio* el día *de hoy* Y para que conste lo firmo.

Carlos Alfonso Erreis

17 Birth certificate of José María Torres, aged 150 years.

to legend, some of the earliest varieties of maize originated here.

Most of the land is a sandy humus, especially in the regions formed by the Chamba and the Uchima rivers—black land originating from thousands of years of silt that has been brought down from higher up the mountains. In the eastern part it is good for cereal agriculture. There are pockets of clay and volcanic ash. The topsoil is about 1.6 meters deep, but in the higher parts it is less deep. In winter, the rivers bring down great quantities of lime, which is put on the fields as an aid to crop production. The higher lands are rich in carbon phosphorous even without the peasants having to burn down the vegetation (their common practice). Away from the paths of the rivers and *wadis,* there is seldom any flooding, as the ground is very porous. There are many bogs and marshes that the villagers would like to see drained and probably planted with sugar cane, but these are the last strongholds of the rare and valuable herbs.

The soil contains calcium; there are calcium, kaolin and gypsum mines in the area. The calcium is particularly good for many kinds of fruit trees—oranges, mangoes, plums, pomegranates, guava, limes, sweet lemons. Cedars, eucalyptus, cachia, camphor, rosemary, avocado, the mango and wilco trees are found in profusion. The condurango tree grows freely on the mountain slopes; it is supposed to prevent and cure cancer: we are at present investigating its properties. The burning of old trees and the planting of new ones is carried out in June. The crop-planting time for the region is August. Most of the villages have nurseries for trees.

On most occasions when I have been there the people's hospitality has extended to giving me medicinal water, which was derived from strips of rough bark, some of which I brought back to this country. Dr. G. Cutler of Kew identified the bark as being from the cascarilla tree, from some varieties of which quinine is obtained. They come in two types in the valley—the Aritusinga and the Cinchona; the bark was of the latter type. The original "Peruvian bark," so highly prized as a cure for malaria before baludrin, first came from this area. The valley is also famous as a healing center for blood disorders, varicose veins, ulcers and heart disease.

The coffee produced here is supposed to be the best in the

whole of Ecuador—it certainly resembles Colombian coffee more than most of Ecuador's coffee. Coffee and sugar grown here are exported. Alcohol is also produced in Vilcambamba—nearly all the villages in the region have their own distilleries. All kinds of green vegetables, cabbages, cauliflowers and celery and legumes, such as peas and beans, are also grown. Important medicinal plants will grow if the land is not cleared for sugar, matico and guayusa in particular, which are regarded as beneficial to the liver and kidneys. In Vilcabamba, they were cutting down trees as fast as they could for their fires, and cutting the hedgerows and small coppices, burning them to make way for the almighty sugar cane that seems to dominate everything. In fact, in this fertile land, with its temperate climate, everything can be grown—from the violet to the fig. But this does not mean that it *is* always grown. More complex agricultural development is often neglected because of an inordinate affection for the sugar cane. Bad cultivation and bad eating habits are the main cause of the troubles that exist in the village (not on the mountain small holdings), where some children actually suffer from rickets—the last disease that they should be suffering from, given the potential of the land. But this is mainly due to the pasta and white rice diet that the village locals believe is part of their Ecuadoran heritage.

In the Quinara river—scenically very beautiful—are found some very fine edible fish (similar to salmon), especially at Tumian Uma, but not much use is made of these by the people, who prefer to obtain half-rotten salt fish from the Pacific.

Above the valley there are bears in the mountains and, in some of the open meadows, glimpses of the tapir may be caught as it heads off over the ridge. The armadillo and tumulla (a kind of spineless porcupine) are found and eaten—cooked by wrapping in clay and putting them on the fire. During the three years I have been associated with Vilcabamba and the region, I have only seen one other type of wild animal—and that was a dead one. It was a species of bandicoot, on the mountainside above San Pedro de la Bendita. In the wilder regions of the sierra there are spectacular bears, tapirs, deer and wolves. There is an unusual bird, called the oven bird, common in the locality. Many of the people like to procure the nest of these birds, and have them as one of the few ornaments that are to be found in their houses.

Domestic animals seem to live a long time here. A dog is said to have reached the age of thirty-seven at Vilcabamba; a donkey was still working at San Pedro at the age of twenty-two the last time I was there—and that is old for a donkey, especially a South American one. Domestic animals thrive in spite of the very hard work that they are put to. But the extent to which such wild animals as deer, tapir, anteaters and armadillos have disappeared, through trapping and hunting, may be an indication of what may happen also to such indigenous plants as the matico—though these have been the last to go in the exploitation of the environment.

This is a region of unique botanical quality. From a medicinal plant point of view, Vilcabamba and its district is the most valuable remaining site of all the villages. The region has a wealth of herbs and is a rich source of interesting plants. During the long years that scorn was heaped by the medical profession on herbal remedies, the plants were even more severely treated in such regions as this. In more progressive regions, with a more flexible attitude toward such methods in the treatment of diseases, many were allowed to survive, but merely as curiosities. But the doctors in the developing countries, such as Ecuador, were taught to be, above all, good conservative doctors, and to approach such things with skepticism. Much of the knowledge of the properties of these plants has already been lost, but some knowledge still remains with the old. Nothing has been written down of this knowledge. This should be done before it is too late.

Luckily the people appreciate the beautiful flowers that grow in the region, and allow them to grow. Also, as they are Roman Catholics, the Virgin's association with flowers helped to protect them further. In the animal kingdom it is quite a different matter. There is war to the finish; domestic animals are exploited in their usefulness to the full, and given little protection from overexertion; wild animals are hunted.

Local legend says that the valley was the true Paradise from which Adam and Eve were expelled. It still retains from that Paradise the purity of the atmosphere, brilliant sunshine and crystal clear sky. It is an area frequented by people who believe it has special qualities, indefinable by normal explanations; thus an "international sage," Dr. Lovewisdom, who lived for a period in a cell on the mountain nearby, referred to "magnetic sunstorms which can eliminate the toxins that cause death—the cell being immortal if it has the means of detoxifying itself." These enigmatic statements are a measure of the air of mystery with which people invest the area. Such ideas have been given as the reasons for the longevity of the inhabitants.

The valley has always been much inhabited. The present village is not the first one to be there—in fact there are signs of two villages pre-dating it, and all around are signs of very early tribes, perhaps nomadic, having lived in the heights above the village. There are extensive ruins of a town or large community in a craterlike valley on the peak of Lambomuna. The ancient village was situated on the lowest slopes of the mountain of Mandango, north of the present village. This was both a pre-Inca and an Inca settlement. The second village was at the confluence of the Uchima and Chamba—very swampy terrain, for which reason it was probably abandoned. Ruins of an ancient convent are still found in this marsh. The early village suffered in addition from an earthquake. The present site is a much more favorable one from every point of view. The church was built there in the middle of the last century.

Southeast of Vilcabamba, on a hill called Surcucunuma, there lies a cemetery in which are buried members of tribes occupying the valley in very ancient times. There are also traces, including broken statues, of a large ancient town. The last of the Inca kings, Atahualpa, was based at one time in the valley of Palmyra, on the other side of Mandango peak, and from there he began his attempts at bargaining with the conquistadores and Pissaro. He eventually went to meet the Spaniards, but they kidnapped him; however, he begged them for his life—saying he would give them all the gold that they desired—and it is said that still, in Lima, can be seen a room with a mark on its walls where the Spaniards indicated to the Incas the height the treasure had to reach before he could be released. It seems that the final amount was slow in coming—some of it from the mines in southern Ecuador. The Spaniards lost their patience and, in a drunken orgy, executed Atahualpa. At that very time it was said that there was a caravan already on its way to Lima carrying gold from the Palmyra district. But when they heard of the murder of Atahualpa they turned back and Quinara, the king's captain, who gave his name to the river that flows through Palmyra, and who was in charge of the caravan and the king's treasures, hid the gold in seven deep burial shafts. It was said that there were a thousand mules waiting to carry the gold to the Spaniards. These treasures included the golden throne of the king, which he took with him wherever he went.

They buried the treasure to make certain that the Spaniards would never get hold of the gold, and marked the spots so that they could one day come back and collect the gold. The main marker, a statue standing about eight feet high, is there to this day on one of the farms in Palmyra but it is thought to have been moved a little. Of course many people have looked for the gold in this region, and there are many deep shafts as evidence of their activity.

One of the Indians who took part in the burying of the treasure happened to fall sick, and went to Lima. Possibly he had malaria. The Jesuits at this time had the monopoly of the quinine bark which was found in the region of Malacatos and which was used to cure the disease. From this Indian the Jesuits found out where the gold was; they obtained a chart from him and set out in an attempt to find the gold. The chart was a sketch map of the place where the treasure was buried, and was made out quite clearly. But they were unlucky—in their haste they overturned the stones and statues which told where the treasures lay, and they were hidden or lost. One Jesuit remained and became deranged and was seen for a few years around the site—always searching but never finding anything; he finally died there.

Two hundred years ago, a fairly poor small holder, Sánchez Orinjana, found on his land a large treasure of gold ingots dislodged by a flood, which was assumed to be from these mines. There were also priceless small ornaments—nose rings, earrings and so forth. He melted them all down, and it took 120 mules to carry the melted-down ingots. These were taken to Quito. Sánchez Orinjana became "marquis" of the area and bought a great deal of land with the money. This is how he became the first Marquis of

Solanda, named after the region in the Palmyra valley where the treasure was found.

At the time of the conquest, Inca puppet leaders held control of the area, but only by the grace and favor of the Spaniards. After this they disappeared and we get no more mention of Inca rulers or of Incas holding office. Their language has now gone and much of their folklore and history has been obscured. From this time on the Spaniards sent viceroys to control the area. One of these had control of the region in which Vilcabamba is situated. The viceroy area of Malacatos is that of Perus Quinine—its name derived from the multitude of quinine trees that grew there. (The wife of the viceroy of Peru was completely cured of fevers from the famous bark brought back from Malacatos in the seventeenth century: the Indians had used this first, and the Spaniards learned it from them.) This region then was given over to the Augustinian Fathers, who were the first missionaries in the region of southern Ecuador. However, all the lands they farmed and cultivated and exploited were later given to Don Ferdinando de la Vega by the King of Spain in 1756.

The region thus has powerful mythology and romantic historical events associated with it. It also has many associations with mystery and sacred qualities. Vilcabamba valley has many sacred places. Among many sacred springs there is the upper spring high up on the ridge of Warango; Petreridos above the village; Tschca-ilomaum (pre-Inca language) Vilca is a spring with much iron, so strong that you cannot drink much of it—people with diseases of the joints, i.e. arthritis, drink it; and on the other side there is the peculiar rock formation of Mandango. At the most conspicuous of these heights there is a cross on the top, called Pinliche Ande. This is one of several crosses mounted on it, and the pupils from the Vilcabamban schools on holy and special days like to vie with each other in leaving one of their personal belongings on top of one of these points to show their prowess at climbing. In the church, there is the grotto dedicated to the Virgin of the Grotto at Lourdes.

San Pedro de la Bendita, not to be outdone, also has its sacred place dedicated to the Virgin, the Virgin of El Cisne, or the Swan (in Spanish). It is a dry, open space high up on the mountains above San Pedro. People who go there see in the distance a swan, but in order to get to it they have to pass around a headland, and by that time the swan has always disappeared. But why should the swan haunt such an unsuitable place for a water bird? (In their daily life the villagers take not the slightest interest in birds. Their philosophy is that God gave them all the animals, including the birds, to eat.)

Interestingly, because of the altitude, and thus the coldness, of these places, Vilcabamba, Nambacola, etc., there are no harmful reptiles there, and although there may be a few snakes, neither we nor anyone we met has ever seen any. Nor are there giant harmful insects, spiders, centipedes or dangerous mosquitoes, or harmful animals.

All this adds to the legend that the area is a paradise, with special and sacred sites. The sacredness of these sites goes back to pre-Colombian times—that is to the time of the Incas, and, who knows, perhaps even before. There are no written histories. All around these villages are signs of prehistoric activities, old village sites, the stones of hut circles and marks on the mountainsides of cultivated fields from days gone by, which are much less rarely found near villages in other areas of southern Ecuador. It is as if, even in those far-off days, these places were set apart and special. Despite the fact that the terrain has been much altered, trees cut down, the plant growth altered, some plants destroyed, and in general rapid and often ignorant changes made, this area still retains its quality of being special, mysterious. It is commented on by visitors and locals alike—there is an extraordinary atmosphere which pervades the region.

We must hope that the discovery of the old people with their remarkable health, and the increase in communications with the towns and cities, does not lead to the exploitation and destruction of these marvelous qualities which make the area such a unique one. There are some signs already that this danger exists—it would be a tragedy if it was allowed to spread.

Having learned something of the plant and animal life of the area, and pursued its history, archaeology and mythology, we began to explore local village life.

5

My First Day
in Vilcabamba

After my first brief visit by bus, I officially announced my presence to the governor of Loja province, Dr. Clotario, by going to visit him. A jeep was put at my disposal and I set off again from Loja to Vilcabamba. There I stayed at the hacienda of Señora Río Frío, above the village.

The day after my arrival I was waked in the early morning by birdsong, the braying of several donkeys and the crowing of many cockerels—sounds that I had not heard in such numbers for years. I was listening dreamily when there was a tap on the door and one of the servants appeared, asking if I had slept well and would I like to accompany the señora to the fields? I thought this was rather an unusual custom, perhaps one that called for caution at such an early hour. The jeep-driver's head appeared above that of the servant around the door and I felt that perhaps there was safety in numbers—and then the señora appeared with a bottle of whiskey in one hand and a bucket in the other. It was the stool in the hand of the servant that made me realize what was afoot; we were going to the field to do some milking. It was, I must admit, curiosity that persuaded me to go along with them, and so the little caravan plus several lean dogs set off for one of the lovely green areas on the slopes of the nearby mountains.

After going through a rather unkempt orange orchard we came to a herd of cows. With the herd were some calves, but the cows seemed not at all bad-tempered, even when Señora Río Frío hit them with the stool and caught one of the calves. The servant went to another and started milking her. Halfway through the milking, the frothing milk was poured into a glass until it was about three-quarters full, and then the whiskey bottle was produced and the glass was filled to the very brim with it, and handed to me. A spoon was brought out of the driver's pocket and the mixture stirred up. I was given to understand that this was one of the more refined of the local drinks. At that time of day I would have preferred one of the more country-style drinks— a kind of sugar-cane drink which ferments later in the stomach. A glass of good spring water is almost unobtainable in those regions unless you climb to the very mountaintop—as the houses are built along the bed of the stream, the water gets contaminated on its way down.

On the way back the señora asked me a host of questions, the majority personal, such as was I married; but others included what I thought of the valley and its people, why had I come all the way from London to see old people—were there not any old people in England? Oh! it was the age of them—were there not people of 120 and 130 in London? Was this so very strange? Some of the questions would not have been asked by any English person even after an acquaintanceship of several months. She also volunteered some information. It was true indeed that many of the oldest people were still working. There was Gabriel Sánchez who was 120, but he was going a bit deaf now; although he was still hoeing his corn on the mountainside when she last saw him.

On our way back we picked some oranges. These oranges plus cafe tinto (black coffee) made up my breakfast for that day. The custom of whiskey and fresh warm milk to drink was obviously a very newly introduced one, no matter what anyone claimed. For one thing, the people in the village down below could not possibly afford a bottle of whiskey even if they saved up for a year. From what I had heard, and what I saw with my own eyes later, they lived mainly off the produce of their small holdings, which only gave them a small income.

By the time we had reached the hacienda the village was awake and from the valley below a blue smoke haze rose above the little white clouds found in the valleys of the Andes. Breakfast was sweet bread rolls, with some kind of jam that looked very much like tomato jam. There was also a hairy cheese (hairy because of too much human handling) which I could not quite stomach at that hour. It was obvious that I had found a useful as well as a pleasant friend, for not only was Señora Río Frío the lady of the manor, but her hacienda was a center for the town, and for country people who were a bit nervous of going into town. It looked as though it would be a good base, and it had a splendid view of the village below.

The driver said that it was possible for him to stay a few days, but if it was to be for a longer period he would have to get a message back to Loja. These things were discussed after breakfast. I learned that usually there were communications with Loja only once a week, so the jeep was going to be very useful—in fact essential, for it appeared that the very old were in the farmsteads higher up in the narrower valleys that led out of the main valley, and the jeep could get up to these, depending on whether the rivers had been in flood or not. At least it was quicker and more comfortable than by burro.

After breakfast was over, we had a conference on the verandah on where to start the day. I walked, together with Victor, a little orphan Indian boy—a Saraguro, with the brightest eyes I ever saw —the driver and my cameras, to the village, along a charming lane that I had failed to appreciate in the dusk of the previous evening. There were more domestic animals now than I had seen previously on this road, let out of ramshackle lean-to sheds, and grazing and foraging for themselves along its verges. There were also small ginger pigs with thick curly hair, wearing a ruff of forked sticks strategically placed, with points to prevent them getting through the makeshift fences and rough hedges that protected the field crops. Numerous friendly donkeys hee-hawed in greeting as we went along. Here and there, too, were fighting cocks, tied by one leg to stakes. They all had a go at us as we passed by, with their enormous natural spurs looking extremely vicious, and strained forward to the end of their strings until we had gone by.

They challenged each other with crows and stares and lifted wings. They seemed to be some Indian game breed very high on the leg and when they were particularly angry they lifted one shoulder, reminding me of the London spiv!

As we approached the village more people appeared. They all greeted us as we passed by with "Buenas días, señor" and a polite bow. The majority of people we passed seemed now to be rather careworn women in their thirties. Old men and children were conspicuous by their absence.

From a side lane we suddenly saw what looked like a moving mountain of sugar cane bearing down on us rapidly. Victor called on it to halt. The large bundle of sugar cane, on its way to the Río Frío's sugar mill, dropped to the ground to reveal a weather-beaten old gentleman in patched clothes and a large panama hat. He took this off as he bowed to us to reveal a head of almost jet black hair, with a little gray at the side. He was very lean and slim, though the smile he gave us was rather toothless. Victor told him that I was a scientist who had come to look at the old people of the valley and then asked him his age. He was eighty-eight. Victor thought this was nothing unusual and was quite blasé about it. With a smile and a nod, rejecting our offers of help with the heavy load that I could hardly lift off the ground, the old man briskly put the sugar cane back on his unbent shoulders and walked on in the direction of the sugar mill. He had probably cut the sugar cane that morning and traveled several kilometers immediately to avoid the sugar juice bleeding too much from the cane—so he must have been up with the dawn. Although he was toothless, his face had not the sunken look often found on Europeans when they have lost all their teeth. There was something almost boyish about him as he continued down the trail with his load.

As we approached the houses of the village we saw several old people sitting out on the verandahs in the sun. These lived in Vilcabamba with their relatives and some were walking about quite briskly. Some of them were introduced to me by Señora Río Frío, who had finished giving the orders of the day to her farmworkers and who followed us down to the village. She seemed very popular with the local people, partly because she owned the only sugar mill in the district—a source both of income and employment.

One of the people to whom she introduced me was Belamenio Carpio; he was a distant relative of Miguel Carpio, a famous old man whom I already knew lived in the village. Belamenio had a stick and did not look too strong, though he had an alert, characterful face. He turned out to be eighty-three years old—not as old as I had expected, though quite proud of himself and his age. He had quite a potbelly, something that I found to be generally lacking among the centenarians. He was, I think, basking in the reputation of his cousin who lived down the road, and hoped that people would mistake him for Miguel. He often appeared later when I was taking surveys of the people of Vilcabamba and seemed to court having his photograph taken on as many occasions as possible.

6

First Investigations

We decided to make the hacienda of the Río Frío family our center in Vilcabamba—from it we could see the village and the smaller valleys leading off from the plain. There was also the very large verandah where we could work even on the hottest of days. The people liked to come to that house on the hill. It was an imposing place, and we were given a large, airy room each. Occasionally one of the numerous dogs, lean and rather fierce-looking, would come in or scratch at the door. The nights were not peaceful; at every sound coming from the valley below there would be a serenade from the dogs, though eventually they became very friendly. The amenities were few but were far better than those of the lodging house in the plaza, where several people shared one tap and there were no windows in the rooms. It was also much too public.

We were going to look at the following groups around Vilcabamba:

> Girls ten to thirteen years old
> Boys ten to thirteen years old
> Teen-age girls
> Teen-age boys
> Women thirty to thirty-five years old

Men thirty to thirty-five years old
Women fifty to sixty years old
Men fifty to sixty years old
Women over seventy years old
Men over seventy years old

These groups were also the ones looked at in the other villages. In this way we covered information from childhood to old age.

There were at least ten centenarians within the close vicinity of Vilcabamba village whom we knew would come in because arrangements had been made by the mayor. We planned to talk to the boys and girls in the schools, with the co-operation of their teachers, and after this to interview the older people at the house of Padre Bravo, as he had a suitable room. Thus a general view of health could be built up. We estimated that the whole program would take about a fortnight in Vilcabamba, perhaps a little less if everyone co-operated, but we were not expecting the wonderful reaction that began on the second day.

We planned that we would visit the schools first, with questionnaires on diet, teeth, habits and physique compiled by Dr. Franks of Birmingham University and myself. From these and the people that we interviewed we hoped to get vital particulars of their diet, daily habits, information on their teeth and the water they drank.

The schools in the center of the village are reserved for girls (about two hundred), the boys being in schools on the outskirts of the village. As we came up the steps of the central girls' school the head teacher was there to meet us, together with some of the members of the staff, all with delightful smiles. Dr. Lolita Samaniego, our doctor, was now with us. All the pupils to whom I hoped to speak were presented in long lines. I gave the reasons why we had come, and what we intended to do, with their help. At this speech there was great enthusiasm from them all. Everyone wanted to be the first to come and answer the questionnaire and to have a medical examination from Dr. Lolita. We carried out one of the teacher's tables and set out chairs on the verandah, which was crowded with aspirants. We had to try to counter this diplomatically, for we could only question one person every twenty minutes. We were really afraid that they might lose their enthusiasm, but as I gave them the used dental mirrors they pressed forward more than ever. Some of those little girls had, I am sure, never seen a mirror before, and showed intense interest in them—in fact there were squabbles over them.

All our surveys, in every age group, were assisted with enthusiasm. We had the help of a young girl, Magdalena, who was very lively and knew how to keep up the spirits of those whom we were interviewing when they were flagging. She was a comedienne in a land of rather glum individuals. The women especially looked tired and careworn.

As far as we know, no similar surveys had been carried out before, at least not in connection with their diet and physique. It became our custom to give a talk to them before starting on the reports. All listened attentively. From the information that the children gave we found out who had very old grandparents; sometimes they would be standing nearby and we would get them talking into the tape recorder together. At the same time we took photographs of them.

We were interested in the family life and sexual habits of the people; also, we wanted to find out whether the difference in the aging process affected menstruation, childbearing capacity, fertility, the menopause and sexuality generally.

The lunch hour came and went, marked by the arrival of many of the elders of the village who had come to watch the scene. Some of the boys brought along some food wrapped in maize leaves. It looked like ground rice and tasted rather sweet; it was delicious, and on inquiring I found that it was made of ground maize and brown sugar.

As we worked on, a strong breeze rose and blew all our papers like confetti. All over the playground they went, and some even over the building. This is what some of the children had been waiting for. With shrieks of delight they chased after them; the dogs barked and scampered behind, the old men chuckled—the children and the ancients were happy together. We made many friends on this day; the stiffness of these people was gone— especially from the elders; we were accepted.

It looked as if the wind would continue to blow, and people started to get restless, mothers calling for their children; some, we knew, had to travel several kilometers. As the sun began to sink and there were only candles for light, easily blown out by the wind, they started to move away. We packed up the paraphernalia of our research, and, feeling very satisfied with our day's work, started back to the hacienda on the hill. At the last house the fighting cocks were still alert and eying each other on the verandah, their eyes bloodshot, still straining at the end of their string tethers.

High tea was waiting—very different from what the peasants in the surrounding hills were having at this moment. There was sweet bread, with black bits in it; jam with black bits in it; masses of whitish, lumpy cheese with black hairs in it; there was coffee with black flies floating on it; lukewarm milk that had been boiled sufficiently to allow one to receive a mouthful of the skin, with a new variety of hairs; and there was meat, of course. The photographer and I were too nervous to ask what the meat was. In fact it could have been anything from the guinea pigs that roamed under the dresser in the kitchen—whose shrill whistles we could hear from time to time throughout the meal—to the little ginger pig that was rubbing itself on the gate as we went out that morning.

As we completed our meal at the hacienda, we saw two small figures in the gathering gloom on the verandah. It was Teresa, a pretty young girl, with her 102-year-old great-grandmother, who had walked the steep two kilometers uphill from their home in the village below. The old lady, María Abarca, moved like a twenty-year-old and it took some persuasion to make her sit down.

7

The Centenarians—
Appearance, Diet
and Health

The villages we investigated, including Vilcabamba, generally have a population of around 750 each, many of these children. Several people of middle years had left due to economic pressures. About half the parish populations were living in scattered small holdings on the surrounding hills and mountainsides, and these were the areas where in general the oldest people lived and were healthy to the end of their lives. Most of the parishioners had some form of contact with each other during the course of the year, so the people in the villages knew where the oldest people lived and where they came from. They came in, usually on Sundays, some traveling quite long distances. Some came only for Mass at Easter or Christmas. These centenarians and their families, on coming to the village, would not return straight away but went to one of the numerous little shops around the plaza, just as people living in the country in England come to London for the day. Of those people who lived in the village, one in four had a small shop of some sort or another, selling some form of refreshment or pasta which was asked for in soup or taken away in packets as a treat. Rarely would the old visitors go into the house itself, but would sit on the verandah, on the roughhewn benches

provided for this purpose. Others would sit on the raised wooden
walk that runs along the outside of the houses like some form of a
wooden pavement.

Everyone will be interested to know something of the appearance and physique of the centenarians. Let us start with a look at
the top of the head, their hair. The majority of the men are extremely hairy. It grows in tufts out of their ears and it is common
to see their bright eyes looking out of a furze of hair. The backs of
the hands, the chests and, of course, the calves of the legs, are covered with a thick matt of hair. The profuse growth of hair on their
heads would delight any teen-ager, but it was often of a very
coarse variety and very dull, like that of a hairbrush or even horse-
hair. I have seen this kind of hair on Orientals, but there was nothing oriental about their features. These features would have been
more in keeping with the Irish or with the peoples from the islands of Scotland; they certainly would not have looked out of
place there. The women's hair was glossy and always in long
tresses—sometimes in plaits. Even in the very old women it was a
blueish color—never white—and there was a great profusion of it,
often reaching down to far below the waist even in those of 110 or
more. They were very proud of this crowning glory and we often
saw these old ladies combing their tresses before their front doors.
There were many herbs that they collected in which to wash their
hair, and it was probably as a result of this refined treatment that
the hair was so healthy. These women were extremely feminine—
there was never the hint of a mustache as is often found on
Spanish women.

About half the population had blue eyes, the rest brown; yet
they did not lose their sight in old age. In our own communities it
is often blue eyes that lose their sight first. They all had beautiful
eyes, strong, arched eyebrows and long lashes; large eyes that
looked at you directly. The centenarians had eyes with a brilliant
sparkle, the blue eyes particularly brilliant; they also had very fair
skins.

In height generally they were not tall, about five feet five inches
on the average. But one would come across some well-grown individuals: Miguel Carpio was, at six feet, the tallest centenarian we
met. The great-granddaughter of Gabriel Sánchez towered above

Sánchez at the age of fourteen. Generally these taller people were remarkably good-looking and when the males were without whiskers it could be clearly seen that the faces were oval. These taller people were perfectly formed, right down to their very beautiful hands. They seemed to retain one or two teeth for longer than most of the people we saw. I think it is here that we get the real centenarian type. Most remarkable to observe were the large, long ears, much more accentuated with the taller people; and the eaglelike long noses that I have seen in no other group of people. This may be due to some of them being descended from the Spanish soldiers, who fought and lost at the battle of Pichincha, or it could be due to them belonging to a race far older than the Incas. The figures and the ceramic art found by archaeologists in southern Ecuador, Colombia and Peru, show just these attributes. The group could have been left in this valley high in the mountains of southern Ecuador, and, through fear, adopted Spanish names so that they and their children would not be molested by the Spaniards. This has been known to happen.

Except for those who had decided to live in the village, obesity among the old people was non-existent, and we only observed one case, a man of 83 of the Carpio clan. They were otherwise all lean, slim and extremely agile. If you were walking behind a man, until you caught up with him you would not know if he was 40 or 120, such was the nature of their walk. There was certainly much passion for life—it could easily be seen, even in the children; but this vitality was found almost exclusively in the mountain population. There was something dynamic—even tigerlike—about their movements, which was even more remarkable as the majority of people only a village away in Vilcabamba were totally or predominantly white people; however, in the remoter regions, they were often Indians, sometimes of the rather unusual Saraguro type.

I wanted to see if there were some people older than Miguel Carpio (123), with baptismal certificates to show their age. This was an essential point because other groups of old people that we know of in the world have no such documents to prove their age conclusively. The existence of these very old people, together with documentary proof of their great ages, showed us that this is a place of great and unusual interest where people live longer, and are healthy to the end of their days—of remarkable interest not only to lay people but also to scientists and medical people the world over. These are the only people whom we can call "age-known specimens" found in the world today.

In the evenings, after we had spent much hard work on the surveys, we visited the very old and some of their families for reports, as I wanted to ask them questions about their family trees. We found that the ages of the old people tallied with what they stated when they talked of their escapades of years ago. For instance, Miguel Carpio said he was 123, and by many cross-checkings with people who had known him as a young man and the times that he had recorded of known dated events—such as the invasion by Peru into Ecuador in 1902—we found him to be certainly no younger; in fact by some calculations he seemed to be 129. What we found very interesting, though, was that the oldest were males, and the number of women centenarians was smaller after the age of 105. I will discuss this later in the project.

The girls were immature for their ages, especially physically. They usually started menstruating at 13 at the earliest; some only started when they were 18. They were also flat-chested up to the age of 18, and this was true of the female centenarians, such as Mercedes Coriva (148 years old). Many young girls, we observed, took an interest in sex at a very young age, often before they were physically mature. They must have been familiar with love-making as they were with the adults during the fiestas—often an opportunity for four days of sexual license. Boys also had few signs of puberty at 11 or 12; on the whole these began to appear at 15 or so.

Childbirth was something which rarely caused death—we found no records of this in the certificates we examined, and certainly there was little evident fear of childbirth. The menopause often arrived much later than we would find in Europe. One of the first women I met, who was with her two youngest sons of 10 and 12, surprised me by saying she was 64—she looked about 35! She saw nothing unusual in her last child having been born when she was 54—and on asking her and others, we discovered that it was quite common for women to go on having children up to the age of 60. Thirty per cent of the live births in the valley were to women of 45 or over, *twice* as many as in the 25 to 34 group.

Sexual mores were presented differently by different people in the community. One of the doctors helping us said the men lived such a "good" life that they lived longer, and had no prostate trouble! But we could not help noticing that some of the centenarians were still notorious for their affairs. Passion is certainly very important to these people and love-making is carried on irrespective of age, the women making the advances as much as the men. It is assumed that every man, in particular, must be having a sexual relationship with someone. It was something of a trial that this included us—so that there were feuds over our suspected favors! The centenarians boasted openly of the number of lovers they could take in one night at the age of 80 onward, and all who had wives said that they made love to them. Some of the older centenarian men might have become temporarily less potent, but this was soon altered with the appearance of a good-looking woman—they were revived as a flower by the rays of the sun! Their descriptions of love-making and attractive women seemed to us very healthy and uninhibited—there was no concept of the "dirty old man" such as we have had in the West. Passion and love were things to be enjoyed at all ages. In Vilcabamba until his recent death at 102, lived Eudoro Guerrero Ochoa, well known and loved among the villagers, who had had seven wives. His sexual escapades with married and single women were legendary—leading to his nearly being shot! But his wit and humor meant that no one was angry with him for very long. Most of the male centenarians have had at least two wives, the second usually about forty years younger than themselves.

Occasionally the married women live to a great age—the Carrions had grown old together, she being 140 and he 145 years old—but normally married women died much younger than the single women. Of the women centenarians we found, very few had been married. Most of the married women over thirty had a tired, rather bedraggled look; they are definitely second-class citizens in relation to the men, and often seemed to be treated as sexual objects, especially on feast days and weekends. They were frequently dull and listless through exhaustion from childbearing

and child rearing. Nevertheless, there was romanticism too, especially among young people—we heard at various times the strum-
ming of a guitar and singing in the early hours of the morning
under the windows of some young women. A few of the married
women were very lively-looking and exceptionally voluptuous.
But these were the exception. And alas, the good looks were
spoiled if the women started to smile, for usually they lost their
teeth at such an early age that even those in their twenties might
exhibit a completely toothless grin!

Our interviews with fifty or so women bore out that their home
life was often exhausting and a burden. Great satisfaction is felt
by men if their wives are pregnant—it is considered a sign of
sexual prowess. The men say they are never happier than when
they can see their women "full" and know it is of their doing.
They talk of their pregnant wives with pride, and comment on
what delight they can get from her each night without any problems of contraception. There was only one married woman over
twenty-five who had fewer than four children—the rest had between four and fourteen. They all had knowledge of the fertility
drug, gayuna, and corroborated what their men had told us—that
it appeared to increase men's drive but to diminish the women's.

One of the natural methods of birth control results from the
women usually breast-feeding their babies for at least two years.
Breast-feeding holds no taboos—it is often done publicly—and
they are proud to show their breasts. There are signs that breasts
have been objects of worship in the region—stone figurines are
found in the niches of rocks, showing sometimes a single breast,
sometimes a cluster. Often when a mother was talking to us and
brought out her breast for feeding we would see a small dark ob-
ject, carved in stone, nestling between the breasts. This turned out
to be a model of an erect penis or phallus. Many of the men also
carried such models, usually larger and made of wood, in their
pockets.

Babies seemed moderately strong at birth, but by their fourth
year only half have survived; the diseases most likely to cause
death at this age were measles and gastroenteritis. As in other
countries, proportionately more girls survived than boys. Although producing children was highly valued by the men, and

their fertility seen as something they could be proud of (the mayor had had twenty-three children, not all legitimate), when we asked them how many children they had they would (with the exception of the mayor) invariably tell us only of their sons. It was only after a lot of questioning that we found out about their daughters as well.

Legitimacy of children was very important in these communities, though there were obviously plenty of extramarital affairs, which the authorities were reluctant to admit to. There were also several couples who were not married but lived together, and some where husband and wife lived separately. Illegitimate children and their mothers often became outcasts and lived outside the community proper, as we discovered during our search for herbs. A rather motley group of people followed us during this search, not generally approved of by the locals or by the Ecuadoran doctor in our party (despite the fact that she herself was divorced, a rare thing in Ecuador). These people turned out to be bastards—many of them children of school age who could not go to school, firstly because one had to pay to go to school, and secondly because few of them would have been accepted because of the stigma of illegitimacy. They could not read or write. Theirs was a simple world. This stigma has existed over several centuries: we found on looking at the village registers (some of which go back to the late sixteenth century) that the word *bastardo* is often seen in reference to the births.

These children were often very bright and smiling; their clothes were faded and patched, and they smiled through the grime on their faces. The "outlaws" lived on the perimeter of the village proper. The huts were occupied entirely by women—we never found out what became of the boy babies. These women were far less inhibited than the villagers, and showed a great contrast with the married women living with their husbands, with their voluminous petticoats of respectability. We supposed that during feast days or at weekends the men would visit these huts and sleep with the women. In fact, even the villagers did not always allow Roman Catholic morality to dominate their sexual lives—often my photographer and I were offered the prettiest of the girls! Yet the stigma of illegitimacy lasted even when people became centenarians. Several of the women, and a few of the men, on our list of centenarians did not come to the meetings arranged by the priests, and when we checked we found they and the priest were no longer in touch for reasons of convention—either because they were living as concubines, or because they were bastards.

There were no fears among the men that tobacco or drugs would create impotence or disease. They smoked and drank freely to the last, though women didn't take drugs. Several different types of drugs were taken, including wilco from the wilco tree. Some of these made them high and not fully responsible for their actions; when in this state they were often seen in a state of stupor at the side of the road, lost to the world, in danger of being trodden on or robbed. The women drank occasionally, but never at the same time as their husbands, so that one partner always remained sober.

We investigated diet very thoroughly, thinking it was likely to be an important factor in their lives and health. It was interesting to see what these rather monotonous diets consisted of and to see the differences in the diet of the folk from the mountain farms from that of the villagers themselves. Here is a list of the items that made up the diet of the mountain people: yucca or cassava (a kind of root that above the ground looks like a small cherry tree, while below the root is gray on the outside and white and brittle on the inside, rather like a parsnip. It is poisonous unless cooked). Then there is maize; much maize is eaten as individual berries, boiled, or as we have it, in the form of sweet corn; potatoes, both cultivated and wild; beans, similar to locust beans, and soya beans. There is also cottage cheese, which is usually made from cows' or goats' milk placed in the paunches of recently killed animals. It is left there for eight days until rennet, an enzyme, seeps into it from the walls of the animal's stomach. This transforms the milk, which is then mixed with orange peel, pressed slightly and presented at table together with pieces of meat. Eggs are eaten, usually either raw or almost raw. Meat is very rare unless one member of the family is a herdsman (more common these days than before). When meat was rarer in the diet, the children of the family were invariably fat; now the only fat children we saw were those who had eaten this earlier range of foods.

In fact, the children sometimes looked thin to the point of emaciation, the girls more so than the boys. Most of the items were cooked. There were also green vegetables, a kind of cabbage, marrows and pumpkins, and fruit.

The most outstanding thing about the physical features of the people, whether from the actual villages or the mountain farms, was that they all had decayed teeth. In most cases all their front teeth had gone by the age of thirteen or fourteen and their grinders (or molars) were just hollow shells. What was the cause of this? When we moved on to study the teen-agers, tooth decay was the norm also. It happened that their teeth were literally dissolving away. The gums were extremely healthy. Losing their teeth at a comparatively early age means that they have to subsist on soft foods and most of the people had a diet that is gruel-based. I asked the old people how they managed to eat, and they indicated—often in most amusing ways and with many mouth openings to show them bereft of teeth—that their gums had become hardened. If the decay was to do with small traces of lead then the gums would not have looked so healthy. The gums in fact would have looked as they do in some forms of periodontal disease, soft and glue-like, and would be bleeding constantly. None of these signs existed. And there is no doubt that they could not have been so lucid at the end of their days if they had had excessive lead in their diet. Even slightly too much affects the brain.

If the gums do harden, so it seems do the muscles of the face, for the people in these villages do not seem to lose the contours of their faces as is so often found in the toothless in Europe. In fact, to have one's teeth extracted is normally the quickest way to start looking old.

Sugar we thought was not the culprit: there was very little of this in their diet. True, as children they often suck sugar cane as a form of sweet, and this was about the only thing they would ever get in this line; but it would be unlikely to be the cause of such excessive tooth rot, especially when there is plenty of information about the children in Southeast Asia who suck on this from the age of three to twenty-three with no obvious decay in their teeth.

One day when business was a little slack the priest, Padre Francisco Bravo, came and said he had something rather interesting to show us in his office, and there on his desk he had a freshly dug up human skull. It still had earth and roots clinging to it. I examined this. It was that of a young woman and from its sutures she could not have been beyond the age of twenty-five. The few remaining teeth in the upper jaw were badly decayed—not by periodontal disease, which is mostly caused by faulty diet—but the teeth were decaying, the front ones nearly all gone and the grinders just shells, as could only occur through the slow destruction of a mineral. The skull was at least three hundred years old. It had been found in an old cemetery at the other end of the village and had been brought to the padre for safekeeping. Now this and others that were brought in from the cemetery indicate that conditions in the area in earlier days were similar to those found now; whatever it was that caused the decay, the owner of the skull must have had a difficult time trying to eat a normal diet, and must have been eating food of a soft nature. It was not the skull of an Indian.

Our request to investigate the diet in some of the isolated farmsteads and hamlets led us to a house in the mountains where we found an old lady and a slim, dark girl. They told us that an old man also lived there, whom we would certainly wish to meet as he was so old, but he was out collecting maize for breakfast. So we accepted their invitation to a meal, and admired the view from the verandah, listening to the cries of many more birds than were seen down in Vilcabamba. Their garden was full of flowers and hummingbirds. I had not seen so many hummingbirds since I had been in South America.

The old man returned in a few minutes with a bag of corn cobs, rather larger than the ones I had been used to seeing in Quito or Loja. They set about boiling these over an open fire and were also preparing other things inside. We did not have to wait long for breakfast: on tin plates came out a slab of curd cheese, several boiled corn cobs, some yucca, some loose grains of a larger kind of corn on side dishes, as well as some small potatoes that looked very much like wild ones, and some soya beans. This made up quite a nutritious meal. We were given some water to drink from the nearby small stream.

The girl was beautiful. Her figure was shapely enough, but something we did caused her to smile and there were almost no teeth there! All the front teeth had gone and there were only the grinders left. I asked the men who were with me about this and they said it was usual for people not to have any teeth after the age of 20—wasn't it the same in England? This sounded interesting. We had a chance to check the mouths of the others; one of the men with us had only one tooth in his entire mouth. The other man, who turned out to be 120 years old, also had no teeth and had had none for fifty years, and yet his face had not shrunk. This seemed to indicate something special about their diet which could also be linked with longevity; it could also be that, having to subsist on gruel from early in life, some internal reaction was perhaps set up which gave their insides little work to do and helped them to live to their great ages. But people have studied so little about diet that it is still not known if the consistency of a diet is of importance to health or not. It is known that a diet that gives the intestines too much work can injure them—such as the diet of our ancestors in the Middle Ages, who were thought to become prematurely old partially through this. But what caused their teeth to go so early in the first place? Was it the same cause that allowed them to remain generally healthy—something harmful to the teeth but good for the body? Sugar was not the culprit: there was very little of this in their diet. In fact, the only thing obviously likely to cause decay that we immediately came across was the locally made rum. We wondered whether a trace element in the water could be affecting the teeth and maybe other areas of their bodies. This we investigated later, and came to some interesting conclusions, discussed in a later chapter.

We continued to pursue our study of the diet in our search for the causes for the prevalence of "super" centenarians in the Vilcabamba mountain district. We thought we might get a more accurate view of the *village* diet, and the general life of the village, if we stayed at the little hotel or boarding house that I noticed on the plaza, rather than stay with the rich people who occupied the hacienda. There were no meals given at the hotel, and we were asked to go to the little restaurant opposite. There we had to wait an hour for the meal and found it not to be very much different from that in the restaurants at Loja. The basis for the meal was the brilliant yellow soup that I had had dished up at Saraguro, an

Indian town a little way from Loja—with the addition there of goats' and pigs' eyes. By some happy accident, they had this time omitted the eyes, but in every other detail, even to the lumps about whose nature we preferred to remain ignorant, it was very similar.

The village people's diet was based on pasta, white flour, white sugar and tinned foods—all much less good for the health than the more austere mountain diet—and the villagers looked, and were, much less healthy. Many of these foods were introduced from the towns.

The food at the hacienda, too, was similar to that which one might get in the town, with the addition of more meat. They seemed to slaughter the pigs in the back garden. From childhood, the villager would be told that pork was the greatest of delicacies and that he was very privileged to eat it. After the slaughter of pigs there is usually a grand cooking session in the kitchen, and an enormous amount of cakes will be made from pig fat. Large helpings of hamburgers are placed on plates, often with their centers not well cooked, and those not used to the diet may well fall ill. I am convinced that if the village becomes more affluent, town habits will be brought in even more—and, with them, more bodily ills.

The remarkable fact about the health of the centenarians is that they hardly suffer at all from killer diseases such as cancer, heart disease and diabetes, and yet in nearby areas and towns these diseases are common. What are the factors accounting for this? We explored the lives of these people to see in what ways they did and did not have health problems, and what contributions their diet, way of life, etc., might be making.

Of course, the reason for the monotonous and austere diet of the mountain people is their poverty. The cause of death among the richer peoples of the world, especially those who have the opportunity of dining on rich food, is very often heart ailments and other diseases associated with unhealthy dietary factors. We definitely found that the majority of those people who lived to a great age did not live in the towns or villages, but on the homesteads and lonely farms in the mountains. They might often come into the towns and villages to die, but otherwise their lives were spent in the mountains.

Since first investigating their diet, I have met Dr. Dennis Burkitt from the Medical Research Center. He told me that while working with many "primitive" peoples, he found that those whose diet was based on beans, potatoes and grain rarely had heart disease or cancer. Perhaps the cancer-forming agents are affected in the stomach from the very start of life by such a diet, so we may have an excellent combination of factors here. There is a possibility which cannot be ruled out that, due to their diet, either large or small parasites in their stomachs may cause some form of protection against debilitating diseases by eating away at morbid matter in which dangerous toxins could grow, such as cancer and diabetes. Some specialists believe that these parasites affect the blood in some way to keep it pure, so that the causes of heart disease may be removed, such as thrombosis and hardening of the arteries. The cholesterol level in the blood of these people is certainly extremely low. The cholesterol often accumulating on the sides of the arteries among other communities seems with these people unable to form. There may be, too, a form of fungi developing and living in the intestines and killing all harmful bacteria that produce impurities in the bloodstream, perhaps at the same time encouraging antitoxins and antibodies. Thus the normal, healthy metabolism of the body is protected. The lack of cancer and heart disease is not necessarily the only reason why people live to be centenarians—but if cancer and heart disease are ruled out in their lives, this obviously gives them a much better chance of survival.

Only within recent years have cattle come to these valleys in any great quantity and those villages that have fewer cattle also have fewer parasites. Amoebic dysentery is endemic; it is passed on through unwashed hands. There are no bathrooms or lavatories in these villages—people use the fields for that purpose. The amoebas survive in the soil; people with unwashed hands prepare the food (often uncooked, like melons and papayas etc.). Thus it is passed on. Once this disease establishes itself it is very hard to get rid of; it is very debilitating, and attacks the liver. After several years this can produce a weak condition—which is sometimes mistaken by outsiders for laziness—as with the Mestizos and their so-called *mañana* outlook. Certainly we found that the majority of the people in the villages have some form of internal parasite, e.g. tapeworm, roundworm, hookworm, amoebic dysentery; and there are various others that are peculiar to these regions. These may be setting up reactions. They do affect the liver and the kidneys: the majority of the two hundred people examined in Vilcabamba claimed that they had troubles in those areas of the body.

Another source of parasites is pig meat. Pigs have been introduced only recently—they are little runts (very few are more than forty pounds in weight), and full of parasites. I had not seen the full havoc that the trichinosis parasites can cause in older people until we were examining some of the older men, and one took off his shirt for examination. On his chest were great furrows, resembling the runs that moles make in fields, six or seven of these going right across the pectoral muscles of his chest. Trichinosis is easily passed on, especially if the meat is insufficiently cooked: for quite a lot of the muscular tissue near the bone can escape proper cooking and the parasites survive.

Many of their minor health problems come from the rivers. I had heard that they used one river for washing and bathing, and the other for drinking only. On closer study, it turned out that both rivers were used for everything, including the cleaning out of cattle's and pigs' paunches several days old. These were then used, with the attendant parasites, for the setting of cheese. Again, many of the cattle and pigs lived their lives near the river, constantly on its banks; wherever these had been there was a danger of hookworm, which could be picked up if the people went barefoot along the paths used by the cattle. These unpleasant parasites make an entry into the body through the sole of the foot, and then work their way through to the liver, to which organ they attach themselves with a hook. They may remain for several years in the body of the host if no treatment is given, with an extremely debilitating effect. The treatment is very simple, but not always seen to be necessary. It is a parasite that often attacks children, and is one of the main causes of potbellies; very few children live beyond the age of four if this sickness goes untreated, because these parasites give off poison.

Yet another unpleasant parasite that anyone can get, visitor or resident, is the sand-flea. It is everywhere, lying in wait on the paths, and if one walks along barefoot one can feel a sharp pain as if stepping on a thorn. These unpleasant little creatures enter through the hole they have made in the foot, where they immediately start to lay their eggs. If the site of entry is inspected after a few days, a very neat circular area can be seen, with some beautiful, small pearly eggs ready to hatch. If it remains neglected, these then hatch out and the infection continues. In better sanitary conditions the majority of these troubles could be eliminated. At present it is chiefly the children who suffer. The small ones often have distended stomachs, and cry continuously; many do not survive their first year, and the church and civil registers are full of records of how they died. Usually the entry just reads: "died of gastroenteritis." If, however, these people survive beyond their fourth year, by which time they have built up a resistance, and then suffer no accident, they usually (if they are males) live to a ripe old age in the tranquil air of these valleys.

Besides parasites, there are epidemics of ordinary dysentery, and this is passed on in the same way. The only way to break the chain of these diseases is through cleanliness. Bathrooms in the houses would certainly help. There would be much to be said for having a hydroelectric scheme, harnessing one of the two rivers (the Chamba or Uchima) at very low cost. My suggestions for introducing bathrooms had a very lukewarm reception—they are expensive, and there are very few per capita in Ecuador. Clean kitchens, so that the food can be prepared hygenically, would also prevent infection.

The herbs that the old were constantly seen to be collecting at the sides of the roads and in the hedgerows were used medicinally, and when we asked what they were used for, the answer was often that they were supposed to be good for the liver or the kidneys and in two cases for the heart. After a few days in Vilcabamba, and many conversations with the old people, it was obvious that we had to take a closer look at these herbs that are praised by so many of the local people as seemingly miraculous cures for all ills. Several of the inhabitants were eager to volunteer their help in this matter.

On the morning of the "herb" day, village life started as usual at about 6:30 A.M. There was already a small knot of people gathered together on the verandah of the hacienda, waiting to conduct us to places where herbs could be collected. The leader of the band was a little old lady, wearing a varnished straw hat with flowers around it on her head. Also in her group were two bright young girls. There was a quiet, middle-aged man standing by himself, who later introduced himself as José Pardo, the deputy mayor of the village.

Our little caravan started off in the general direction of the river, passing through a charming orange grove and a half-cut field of sugar cane. One of the little girls, among the prettiest that we had seen in Vilcabamba, was striking for having the typical features of the locality—the characteristic large nose and long ears, and typically oval face. Dr. Samaniego was accompanying us and I asked her to inquire of the little wizened woman with the girls who this pretty child was. She turned out to be the old lady's niece. She also had a great-grandmother of 102, whom we later talked to at the hacienda. This girl was called Teresa and could not read or write; the family had not the money to send her to the village school. We later found this was the situation for many children in the area. School was neither free nor cheap.

The old lady pointed out all the herbs, and picked the surface plants, but it was generally left to the two girls to act as "pullers" of plants of the deep-rooted variety. These last were often used in herbal remedies. Dr. Samaniego knew quite a lot about these plants. She pointed out one, yopa, with reddish veins in its leaves, and remarked that it was known to be very helpful in cases of heart disease; people used it as a preventative and those people who came to the area already with heart disease used it also; it was an "export" from the valley. I collected some of the seeds for later study. Another type had outstandingly white veins, but medically was not quite so useful in cases of heart disease. Condurango was used as a preventative for cancer, matico for kidney and liver complaints, and gayuna for the heart and fertility—it is said to increase the fertility of women and desire in men, and is much used. It is also planted in the fields to increase the fertility of cattle, which it apparently does very effectively. There were herbs for the hair (matico), for the skin (linka), and for insomnia. It was obvious that herbs were also used to combat stomach and intestinal troubles. Plants of the morning-glory species and the wilco tree can produce hallucinatory drugs—very famous among the Indians.

Then there were herbs used simply for taste, as in tea. Many were used for seasoning the rather frugal fare, rather as we use mint and horseradish for seasoning. There were also some hot peppers that were not generally considered beneficial to health, and were frowned on by the doctors. It became obvious that the older indigenous villagers relied much on herbs in their daily lives.

The plants were encouraged to grow in all sorts of odd places, even in plots on the sides of the road. Partly, I was told, this was because the people who had recently come to live in Vilcabamba neglected the herbs; these people usually were there for their health, or, if they had land, to grow sugar cane and get rich quickly. They would stop at nothing to grow this crop, and would pay the villagers ten sucres a day (about twenty pence) to clear the land for the planting of the ubiquitous sugar cane. Hence the need for herbs to be planted anywhere where the planting of sugar cane was not feasible.

Here is a list of plants, with the ailments they are said to cure:

Yopa: Heart and circulatory problems. There are two varieties, a white and a red-veined type.

Curuba: Kidney and bladder ailments.

Parica: Skin blemishes.

Huilca: Baldness.

Cibil: Internal parasites.

Hatax: Smallpox and other fevers.

Quebracho: Dysentery.

Zumaque: Venereal diseases.

Matico: Diabetes.

Gayuna: To aid fertility.

Condurango: Cancer.

Cedron: Blood purifier.

Ebana: Goiter.

Jataj: Ulcers.

Pariala: Eye troubles.

Bohoba: Rheumatic troubles.

Wilco: This will cause trances similar to those caused by LSD as well as hallucinations.

Aimpa: Blood pressure.

Giola: Rickets.

Cascarilla: The prevention of aging.

On the way back from the herbal excursion (when we learned, with sadness, of the death of José David of influenza, who was reputed to be the oldest person in Vilcabamba), we called at one of the houses for some cedron, the herbal tea that tastes and looks like the best Russian tea, perhaps with a dash more lemon in it. The old lady of the house made another drink, by pouring water on some strips of dried bark from the cascarilla tree of the cinchona variety, a cousin of the tree that produces the quinine bark. This tea had a bitter, but not unpleasant, taste. On inquiring where this bark came from, the lady indicated that it grew far from the village, up on the mountainsides, where they say the old town once stood.

Because of overpopulation, the local inhabitants are trying to use every bit of land for food. This means chopping down many trees and hedges, including sweet lemons, limes and oranges as well as trees providing dyes and laxatives in previous times. These trees may well have contributed to health. And this land clearance means a loss to plant life, including the many fascinating herbs which become more and more rare. People in the villages ask for pills increasingly to cure their ailments. Sadly, the young there regard herbal cures as just so much superstitious nonsense, and their use is disappearing fast. But the mountain people still cure almost exclusively by the use of herbs.

As I have stated, up to the age of four children are the victims of many different diseases—measles, diphtheria, influenza and others. As if this was a blanket protection, they become extremely healthy after this, except for parasites, which afflict children as well as adults. Out of about three hundred children that we examined, not one was deformed or was suffering from more than the side effects of parasites. However, in the towns, like Loja, there is much hepatitis and diabetes. Influenza, which seems to be rife throughout the population in the villages, may strike at any time. During the surveys, when we asked the people what diseases they had had, the answer was always—influenza. It is, I am sure, endemic.

What is so striking to doctors is the suppleness of the centenarians' muscles, which are as good as those belonging normally to people half their age: sometimes the men of a hundred or so had muscles as flexible as a thirty-year-old! There are no general signs of senility. The only way that they may be incapacitated is from the internal parasites, and those in the mountain retreats seem to suffer far less from the side effects of the parasites than the people who live in the villages themselves. There are, of course, plenty of chances for accidents, for hazards are numerous in South America, mostly because of the dangerous roads and driving. It would be interesting to see how much longer even than their present ages they might live if these risks, together with influenza and parasites, were diminished.

As we have said, here in the Andean mountains there is little heart trouble, and those who have been brought up here do not develop it even if they go to live elsewhere. Living at high altitudes is normally thought to produce heart trouble. It does enlarge the heart. And yet, remarkably, the effect is not deleterious to the local inhabitants. Europeans who have lived in the sierra for several years, and have gone for a medical check after returning to Europe, have found themselves in intensive care units before explaining in which part of the world they have been living. For they will have developed hearts often twice the size of normal to allow for the extra exertion of pumping the blood and meeting the body's oxygen requirements at that height.

When we investigated the blood pressure of some of these old people, we found more often than not that they have a blood pressure commonly found in people forty years younger in Western countries. This was true of Miguel Carpio, Dolores Aguirre, Pastos Abaca, Francisca Guaman, Gabriel Sánchez and Rafael Gualen, among many others.

The large calves often seen in their legs may also have devel-

oped to assist in the extra pumping of the blood required, and not
entirely from exercising their legs in the mountainous terrain of
their home region—though many mountain peoples have these
large calves. This phenomenon can be seen as close to home as
Switzerland, farther afield in the New Guinea highlands and
among the numerous tribes in the foothills of the Himalayas.
Physiologists think that such calves may act as second hearts.

It could, of course, be argued that there are antibodies in their
blood that resist the killing diseases such as heart disease and
cancer. This is not known at this time, but their diet, the parasites,
and a lot of exercise may be important in making one or both of
these diseases very rare.

The significance of these villages in the highlands of southern
Ecuador is threefold: not only do people live long, but they do not
get killer diseases, such as cancer, heart disease, diabetes—obviously these are connected. But, on top of that, their old age is
agile, lucid and active. These facts must be seen in association
with the fact that in the nearby towns, such as Loja, these diseases
are rife—sometimes endemic (such as hepatitis). Cancer and heart
disease are both found in large numbers; and there are no centenarians in these towns. The phenomenon of these healthy centenarians is an extraordinary one in many ways.

It is in the high mountain valleys that the true Shangri La, as far
as old age is concerned, is to be found. And the mystery of the
mountains is no new phenomenon. These people often lived to be
over a hundred years old at least as far back as two hundred years.
Other phenomena go back a long way also—the skulls of comparatively young people who lived and died there four hundred years
ago had all lost their molar teeth in exactly the same way as
today's inhabitants.

When the centenarians from the mountains move into the villages because they want to be closer to their younger relatives,
their contact with the much less healthy, more deficient town diet
affects their health. Even symptoms of diabetes may appear. They
still survive to remarkable ages, but they are more decrepit than
the centenarians remaining in the mountains. And the centenarians have almost always spent most of their earlier lives on
their small holdings outside the villages.

We have made much progress in the West. Infant mortality has been cut hugely over the last seventy or eighty years. In England the Health Service means that even people with little money can be assured of treatment for illness. But we have not coped with the problem of old age. The old have not had a proper place in our Western civilization in recent history, and old age here is accompanied by poor health and lack of agility. It is in the fact that these Ecuadoran old can take so active and lucid a part in life that their fascination lies—most of us would like to live long, but only in good health.

In our own Western communities, if a man dies at fifty it is usually one disease that has killed him; if at eighty, he may have eight or ten potential killers in his body; but with these centenarians, such diseases are absent, and the people die either as a result of accidents, or the body just "wears out." We must take care that, in looking at them and their lives, we recognize their immunity and protect them from losing it; we must protect them from the exploitation of repeated "experiments" and "tests"; and we must resist the danger of over-researching—and too many pills and too much medical attention for those unused to them. Miguel Carpio was operated on at the age of 120 for a benign hepatic tumor—a totally unnecessary operation—and it is remarkable that he survived it, though he has now to walk with a stick.

If these centenarians had been found twenty years ago, or even ten years ago, I think they would by now have been exploited out of existence. For the world was not ready to receive them then, and there was not sufficient interest, as there is today, for their reception into the world of science. The general consciousness and knowledge of people today is such that we now accept vegetarianism at least as a normal possibility for a diet. The concept that diet profoundly affects people's lives is acceptable with more groups of people now—far more than fifteen years ago. In the last few years there has been much study of the genetic aspects of old age, and also increased interest in the environmental aspects. Not only are men of science and medicine interested, but so is a great portion of the public.

Now that so many of us live longer, the quality of our lives in old age is of huge importance. This is the preoccupation of many people and the particular interest of the gerontologist. But we are also interested in immortality—this has always been a human preoccupation. And we are fascinated by any hints of it. The urge to discover the "secrets" of the centenarians of the Andes is a strong one. We should learn from these people, but not, in the process, destroy their way of life.

I could see that although we had had such excellent co-operation from the local people in Vilcabamba and its surroundings, had completed the surveys in time and had got well ahead with the other work, such as the taking of samples of soil and water, it was becoming necessary to take a look at the other villages in the vicinity or even farther afield to see if there were any other areas quite like that around Vilcabamba. It would only be after some comparisons that we would be on the path to finding out more about these mysteries and obtaining a more complete story of life in the mountains of southern Ecuador.

8

The Discovery of Other Centenarian Villages

Could the phenomenon of longevity be confined to this one valley? I felt when we were examining the diet question that we should try to find out the extent and the direction that it took, for we were due to take a look at the surrounding villages to see if their diet differed; we could look into their ages at the same time. Did the phenomenon exist outside Vilcabamba—and, if so, did it run north or south, east or west?

Vilcabamba lies almost south of Loja and the winding road took us through mountain passes for forty-five kilometers; then we descended into Vilcabamba valley, which lay like an enormous starfish in the mountains. It was difficult to get over the high mountains that enclosed it. If there were other areas with centenarians, they were beyond these mountains. The only way to get behind them, according to the maps, was to go back to Loja and take the road over Cajamarca mountain.

There had been several signs of vested interests shown among the people of the region and in Loja. Many of the richer people had weekend houses halfway to Vilcabamba—smart little houses situated behind high trees and hedgerows of their own. There was also an idea, understandable under the circumstances, of turning the place into a health spa; it would be to the detriment of most of the people but to the benefit of certain wealthy persons in the village. Many people had told us that there was something afoot, and such a thing, we felt, could ruin the village. All these factors added to our feeling that we should look at other villages, and that in these circumstances it would be as well if we found another place where further studies could be carried out. So far, no one had found any other areas where there were centenarians living—and it was possible that we might find a place even more remarkable than Vilcabamba!

I was reluctant to send in any report to the authorities, and put off the problem of the request that we join in a project for the village. I left the team for a while and returned to Loja. Here I was introduced to the rector of the university and we discussed

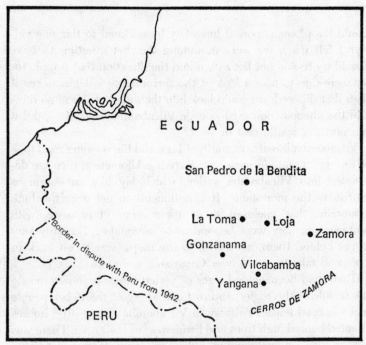

Villages where centenarians in southern Ecuador live.

the problem. He introduced me to a young sociology lecturer who had just returned from Chile, who said that he would be delighted to accompany me in my search for other villages. We went about this work as quietly as possible, for we did not know who was pushing forward the idea of the spa at Vilcabamba, nor which particular big business was involved.

We were loaned the university jeep, and first we went deep into the interior, but found nothing much in the places closer to the hotter areas of jungle; but about one and a half hours beyond Vilcabamba we found the hamlet of Palmyra. Here we met Gabriel Brazo, who was 120 years old, surrounded by hordes of excited children. He was an owl-like little man wearing a knitted cap. When we asked him to take it off his wife took it off for him; underneath he had an excellent head of hair. He had all his faculties, apart from being very slightly deaf. He was squatting on the ground repairing one of his sandals when we met him, and was not at all disturbed by our entry into his domain. He was exceedingly bright and amusing, keeping all the Ecuadorans who were with us laughing, and he provided us with some refreshment. He had the long nose and the long ears of the Vilcabambans. His wife was about 70, and other members of the family were also there; his great-nephew of 49 acted as spokesman to the party, and he had some very bright children who listened to everything being said. This village, about two hours' drive in the jeep from Vilcabamba and the closest of the villages where more centenarians were later found, is, I think, closely linked in other ways with what I term the "centenarian crescent" of Ecuador.

The next day Señor Numa Reinoso (the young lecturer) and I started out in the jeep and crossed over Cajamarca mountain to a place called La Toma. Here, we had heard, there were some old people. When we arrived at the house where they lived the old man there was getting his guitar down from the wall and treated us to a tune. This was Ricardo Aguirre. But he said his family and he had not lived there all their lives. He was a very great age and was living in a very poor house. The padre of La Toma who was our informant said his baptismal certificate was in San Pedro de la Bendita and would I go there, as it was only twenty minutes up the road in the jeep—in fact the next village. Here we met the priest Angel Soto, who was quite an unusual man, dressed in his cassock of course, but wearing a French tammy. He started by handing us a glass of very fine brandy. Out came the books from the dusty old cupboards and from one of the twenty or so registers we found the name of the old man Ricardo Aguirre in the register for the period 1800–50. He was born on 30 June 1842. This made him 131, the second oldest person with an authenticated baptismal record living in San Pedro. The oldest centenarian we came across was Samuel Rochas, born on 20 January 1842, living in San Pedro also. The church records indicate that he is the oldest authenticated person in the world. We photographed the date but doubted if the photo would come out in the dim room. The priest said he would look for others, and would sort through the records. These two have since died: the oldest man is now Francisco Camachot of Sacapalca, born 18 April 1847.

He asked us if we had ever heard of Nambacola, which lay along a road off from La Toma, and suggested we go there with a guide from La Toma. We arranged to meet him in about ten days' time to collect further information, and I also told him that I would like to see the records of any person who had died at a great age. He said he would lay these out on the tables so that they could be filmed and photographed on our return. This called for another glass of brandy all around. By this time the area of the priest's house had become very crowded with sight-seers. We started to return down the corrugated road to La Toma, but just as we were leaving he said: "Take your meat with you if you go, for they have none there." We did not know quite what he meant but we were soon to find out.

By the time we reached La Toma it was too late to set out for Nambacola, so we went back to Loja. The following day we took the jeep and crossed back over Cajamarca mountain to La Toma where we picked up a guide who told us that Nambacola, the place the priest had mentioned, lay one and a half hours away by jeep along a very rough road. He indicated that he, too, was interested in coming along, just for the ride. As we bounced along the corrugated road the driver pointed out the spot where the vehicle that we were in had once somersaulted three times.

After a short while the countryside began to get more arid as the road took us higher, and we left behind us the beautiful green fields, with their silver irrigation pipes. We were now in an area of cactus and trees whose trunks looked much like that of the elephant—strange trees with very thick bases for the storage of water such as are often found in Africa. The trees had started to become flat-topped, which one also sees in other dry arid regions. It was beautiful country, and reminded me of the cultivated parts of the Galapagos Islands. We climbed quite a way up the wide, hanging valley, then turned off on to a much poorer road that would hardly hold the jeep. The soil all around now was a vivid red, but not the usual poor laterite tropical soil. Scattered throughout this area, as if a giant had been playing skittles, were enormous boulders; in some cases people had used them to make the fourth wall of their houses. We had to abandon the jeep for the last kilometer. On arrival at the plaza in the center of the village there were hordes of children. Many of the people here were said by our informants to be living at starvation level.

We met the mayor and the *teniente político,* who, on our inquiries, told us that the rumor was correct—they did have some very old people living in the region, including a man of 145. This man, Señor Carrión, had a wife who was 140, but there was no official records for them. The mayor drew a plan of where the couple could be found; the area was called Piedras Blancas, which was on our way back to La Toma. He added that he would make out a list for us from the civil registers, and would have it ready if we could return in a week's time. He seemed to be acting on behalf of everyone, for the priest was away and they did not know when he would return.

We found the man who was to show us the way sitting with a startlingly beautiful blue-eyed blonde; we all wondered what she was doing there, for blondes are very rare in that region of the mountains. He led us about eight kilometers along the road to the old couple's house. We saw someone outside; our guide hailed him and asked if the old people still lived there. The reply was that Señor Carrión and his wife were at home and they would be pleased to see us. The house was the usual type for these parts, made of adobe, with pantile roof and a rustic verandah. It was on the butt end of a hill and in a very open place; no trees grew here.

We had to wait a little while for the couple to emerge. They certainly looked very old when they appeared but we had only the report of the village chief on their ages. They only did the lightest of work around the homestead. Señor Carrión could see, hear and speak quite well; he could also read. He had been given pills by local doctors recently—he looked rather under the weather compared to some of the old men of San Pedro or even those of Vilcabamba. He insisted on wearing a woolen cap, though he had a good head of hair when it was taken off. We took some pictures of the couple.

We returned to Loja after going up and down the mountain once more. The village of Nambacola was a little way off one of the routes into Peru, two hours' drive from Gonzanamá, the capital of that area. We returned to Nambacola after a week to collect the lists of the old people. We found the *teniente político* waiting for us in the store below the office, with several bottles of beer. It was old beer, but how beer came at all to such a god-forsaken place was beyond our imagination.

As we drank his health we admired the rugged scenery outside, with the mules and the horses tied to the rails amid the dust. The village was in a very beautiful setting, but very dry. It was on a kind of shelf and the broad valley gradually dropped away below until one could see the vivid green of La Toma with a backdrop of blue mountains behind. We also admired the plaque on the wall in Spanish, which read, translated, "Oh, put my spurs upon my breast, my boots and saddle tree, and when the boys lay me to rest, so set my horses free."

By five o'clock the lists had been completed of the old of that village. We were told that many of the people were baptized in the village of Gonzanamá, fifty kilometers farther on. In this region the temporary border with Peru becomes a fingerlike projection, and Gonzanamá lies at the end of this, but it is still considered to be the territory of Ecuador. We stayed the night at Nambacola and went on to Gonzanamá the following day, which meant going back on to the main road. It was strange, fascinating country we passed through. At Colca we found 30 people over 70 out of a population of 300. Then we stopped at Mollepamba where we met an old woman called Carlamanga reputed to be 127, who attributed her age to the water of the region.

At Gonzanamá, there was a large plaza. We entered the large and ancient church with twin towers, where we met the priest coming down the aisle in his cassock and beret. We approached him and he told us that there were plenty of registers and they were all housed in the vestry of the nunnery, where he then took us. The nuns welcomed us with smiles, took us into the vestry, and when we had stated our request three of them got down to work to search in the books. The verger appeared, and the priest gave him a key to a hidden chamber; after a few minutes he returned, covered in dust and weighed down with heavy, ancient-looking books. He put them down in front of the padre on one of the tables. On searching through these interesting documents we found that one was dated 1655, and the names were still quite readable. This established that there were Spanish people in the district by that date. We asked the nuns, led by Madre Superior Madres Dominicas, for their assistance in looking through a dozen or so registers, to see if any of the names of the villagers on our list were there with dates and baptismal records; we also wanted to find any of the death certificates of the very old people coming from the district.

We broke off our search to allow the nuns a little time to study the records, and visited one of the cake shops which had excellent doughnuts. On our return we were pleased to find that they had come across several centenarians actually living in the town. Don Camillo Veintimilla, who was 103, would be found at a house not very far from the market place. We left the nuns to follow up the research and found Don Camillo walking quite briskly in the market. We asked him if the other centenarians whose names we had, all between the ages of 100 and 110, Abel Onevedo, Carlos Ojeda and Lynacio Leon, were at hand. We were also told of two small hamlets that had groups of centenarians. These were El Carmen and Santa Barbara and lay at a lower altitude of about 1,500 meters, very similar to the altitude of Vilcabamba.

We returned to La Toma very satisfied, with a list of villagers. There we received a further message from the padre of San Pedro. He had been looking through the registers and had found many things of interest to us. We went quickly up to San Pedro and, as if expecting us, there was the priest on the steps of his church. The usual ritual of drinking brandy followed—a more local brew this time—and he showed us all the extremely helpful work he had put in with his aides during the week or so that we had been away. We spent the day taking film of the documents. Some of the books here went back to 1708. But for the study we were doing, the book going back to 1820 was the one we required. The padre, with his colleagues, had attached slips of paper, neatly typewritten, to all the entries of great gerontological interest, and it was often striking how even very old records were still beautifully clear. We found even older registers in these places than in Vilcabamba.

We had heard at Loja that there were no Spaniards in the district before about 1820; it was Indian country, they said, until the battle of Pichincha (about 1819) where the Spanish forces were beaten by the Ecuadoran national forces under Simón Bolívar. Some of these Spaniards went to Vilcabamba and some to Loja, then a small village. The population of Loja was later augmented by colonists from Cuenca, a very old Spanish-style city two hundred miles to the north. But these registers indicated otherwise, for all the names were Spanish, except for those in Nambacola. I have since looked up many records of Loja, and it seems that Loja was settled at a much earlier date, probably by 1540. There is a little Spanish colonial church dating from these times.

We found, after much traveling, that the villages in these highlands of Ecuador—the sierra—which have these very old inhabitants, are within closely defined boundaries. Now, after a few weeks' research, we had found eleven villages in whose vicinity lived significant numbers of centenarians, six of them arranged in a crescent shape if seen from the air: Palmyra, Vilcabamba, Nambacola, La Toma (the largest one and really a town), Piedras Blancas and San Pedro de la Bendita; the others, Santa Barbara, El Carmen, Gonzanamá, Mollepamba, Colca, were all close and slightly to the west of this arc.

The positions of these villages are most interesting. Vilcabamba is in a hollow in the mountains where five valleys converge and, seen from above, looks like the arms of a star, Vilcabamba being in the center of this. Nambacola is at the top of a long, hanging

valley, with a wonderful, distant view of a very fertile green plain
—La Toma. La Toma is green, not because it has much rainfall,
but because many rivers come down from the mountains to that
spot. San Pedro is a sort of natural amphitheater, a half circle set
into the side of a very high mountain. Colca, Mollepamba and the
hamlets of El Carmen and Santa Barbara are all in sheltered areas
in the mountains at about the same height above sea level as Vilcabamba—about 1,500 meters. Most of the sites have a
dreamlike quality about them. The weather is superb, and when
walking near San Pedro one suddenly comes across white and red
clover, docks, stinging nettles, plantains, groundsel and many
other common English plants and weeds. The fields, often with
stone walls around them, and the hedgerows with their rambling
roses along the meandering lanes, also have that special English
quality.

Of all the villages in the arc where centenarians are found, Palmyra has the most beautiful setting: its valley is sometimes called
El Dorado. The approach to it is fascinating—there is a very
strong sense of the mysterious; it is here that the captain of Atahualpa, the last of the Inca kings, buried his treasure, or so the
legend goes, so that the Spaniards would not find it.

Why is it so beautiful? It is a region of needle-pointed mountains, seen very clearly through the crisp, pure air. If one goes
through the pass to Vilcabamba, there are many beautiful gorges;
it is an area well wooded, which is unusual for this region, where
many trees have been chopped down in the past. There are sud-
den open spaces, green meadows and then the most wonderful
series of panoramic views as you rise over ridge after unfolding
ridge.

There is no direct contact between the villages in the main crescent, except for Palmyra with Vilcabamba, and La Toma with San
Pedro. If we start down from Palmyra and Vilcabamba, the next
village in the group is Nambacola. The mountain systems are too
complicated for any direct connection by road to Nambacola. In
order to get there, in fact, one has to go back to Loja and this
means crossing over a mountain 2,500 meters high, to La Toma.
This village lies in the hollow at the foot of the mountain. From
there, one gradually climbs upward on a winding road. For the

first ten miles there are lush fields of sugar cane on either side. Soon these are left behind, and the desert scrub takes over. It is here that Nambacola district starts, and with Nambacola and San Pedro the main crescent is completed.

The great range of mountains that lay between Vilcabamba and Nambacola stopped any easy communication that would have suggested some genetic links in the population. Apart from this, the centenarians we encountered had at least three different racial origins. (Genetic bases are also made more doubtful by the northern area, where centenarians are locally reputed to be found in the Ambuki district, little studied at the present time of writing.

We found that San Pedro had been cut off and isolated in a similar way to Vilcabamba until about ten years ago. But the authorities then pushed the main road through it. There was no reason whatever for the road to pass through the village belt, and the result has obviously been to change the nature of life in the village. The old ways have begun to die and much has been lost. The tendency to destroy the rare and the precious is remarkable. Since then similar events are occurring in Vilcabamba, and without care and concern for these remarkable communities they will die. To preserve the good and important qualities to be found there requires the desire to do so, as well as careful planning.

At each village there seemed to be different racial or physical types, so I examined these one by one. The Palmyra people were very similar to the Vilcabambans; their noses were not quite the size of the Vilcabambans', but they had long ears and were about the same height. We need not be surprised at their resembling the Vilcabambans, since as the crow flies Palmyra and Vilcabamba are quite close and constitute the lower part of the crescent.

The Vilcabambans were obviously of very old stock. Some Ecuadorans thought they were white Indians who had quickly adopted Spanish names and customs so that they would not be destroyed by the conquistadores—hence their capacity to survive in the remote Vilcabamba valley. They often had blue eyes. But there are very few Indians here with blue eyes. Many had distinctive long ears, referred to earlier, enormous beaked noses like eagles, and very pale skins. Some, of course, have intermarried with Indians now. Yet they could be the descendants of the rem-

nant of the battered Spanish armies left over from the Battle of
Pichincha. At Nambacola they were nearly all Indian. At La
Toma they were of the coastal type of Mestizos—brown-skinned
people, warm, and much more vivacious than the other people of
the region. At San Pedro, they were chiefly Spanish, had much
broader faces than the Vilcabambans, smaller noses and usually
smaller ears. Vilcabamba, Palmyra and Nambacola were inacces-
sible until recently. Colca and Mollebamba were easy of access.

One of the villages with the oldest people (some of over 130
years of age, and, according to the records, having the most very
old people) is San Pedro de la Bendita. These are the oldest *recorded* people who have ever lived as far as we know. The
churches' records are probably accurate: some of the records giving the ages of people go back to 1840, and no one was seeking
sensation for tourism at that time, high in the mountains of southern Ecuador. On the contrary, they were trying to keep people out
because they had the monopoly of Peruvian or quinine bark and
wanted no visitors there at all. Now the descendants of these people are living in a village through which passes one of the main
roads to Guayaquil, the biggest town in Ecuador, and the coastal
road to Peru!

Environmentally, these eleven areas have much in common.
They have much in common even with Ambuki in the north,
where there may be other centenarians. Diet and climate and the
state of health of the centenarians are important similarities.

We had come across something very important and interesting.
Here we had found not one, but a considerable number of villages, close to which lived these centenarians: the original crescent of these hamlets stretched sixty or more miles, and the
various hamlets were separated from each other by rivers and
high mountains. We had to consider all the possibilities for centenarians being found in this remote area. Could it be that this
region and others have characteristics in common which are the
key to the secrets of longevity? We investigated the significance
of some form of genetic factor; tranquillity and lack of stress in
daily living; temperature; humidity; trace elements in the water
and soil; diet; lack of animal fats; altitude; race; herbs and the
position of the area close to the Equator. We came to some impor-

tant and fascinating conclusions, which we discuss in Chapter 10. Meanwhile, we continued to try and build up a picture of life in these villages and the nearby small holdings, in order to investigate some of these factors further.

9

Life in the Villages
and Mountains

Life in these villages is not packed with excitement: it is serene, and this may be a factor in a long life, for there is little to destroy the equilibrium of the villagers' lives. If you ask one of the older inhabitants what is the cause of such a long life the usual reply is that it is due to the *tranquilo* of the village—the tranquillity of life. Even the climate is never stormy; most of the rain comes at night in both San Pedro and Vilcabamba. Everything is very regular, the temperature keeps to a steady 19° Centigrade, humidity is constant and it gets light and dark at exactly the same time each day of the year, as the area is almost on the Equator.

Ninety per cent of the houses are made of adobe (*tapia* in Spanish) and most of the houses are painted white and have a red tiled roof. There is no efficient lighting system in Vilcabamba. Although some of the houses are wired for electricity, no use was made of this during the three years that I have been associated with the place. Technically, electricity was due to arrive through connections with Loja. In San Pedro, the lighting seemed to flicker, and depended on the water flow through the system. Again, even when there was electric light it was too dim for reading; and as often as not there was no light at all. Few people stayed up after 8:00 P.M. so they certainly had plenty of sleep. In fact one could say they slept nearly half their lives away. The other villages we visited were too remote for any form of electric lighting. The lucky ones had a storm lantern, but most of the lighting was by candle. There are few chimneys—smoke has to make its way through the doors or the pantiles, which is one of the reasons why the interiors of the houses are so black and dark, and why the doors are always open if the occupants are at home.

Vilcabamba has twelve straight streets, crossing each other at right angles. The little streets of the village are at all levels and this means that the gentle slope on which the village rests appears as an unbroken wall of pale red from a distance. One could see that it had been planned properly in 1852, when the present village was built. The streets are wide and unpaved, with room for spacious verandahs. The people make full use of these wide ways to tether the occasional pig, goat or donkey for the night, and they use these places as public lavatories. There are also boulders and some rubbish; there are no dust carts.

Vilcabamba has a lot of little craft shops—cobblers' and blacksmiths'—usually on the corners. Many of the large yards at the back of the houses are used for drying coffee beans and keeping domestic animals. For although the neighboring country of Colombia is noted for its coffee, only the coffee that is grown around Vilcabamba is considered of any quality in Ecuador. The verandahs of the houses, when not occupied by the people sitting and gossiping, are the parade grounds of the tethered fighting cocks. Otherwise there is peace and a striking lack of tension in the town.

Most of the village life revolves around the plaza, a particularly beautiful square in Vilcabamba, and each plaza usually has a very pretty garden in the center. In Vilcabamba the flowers always seem to be marigolds, but in San Pedro there is a variety of flowers. The Vilcabamban gardens have many walks and shady places to sit in. There is a great radiancy, with the golden marigolds, the bright, honey-colored church, the light-colored streets and houses. They all seem strongly to reflect the sunshine; in some cases it was necessary to use a filter when taking photographs.

In most of these villages, one side of the plaza is taken up with the church, the priest's house and offices; there are several stone-tiled steps leading up to the plateau where stood the priest's offices and house, with the church door always open. Where in England there is often a churchyard, in these areas one finds the priest's garden plot, for he generally has a few fruit trees, a yard for hens, ducks (usually Muscovys) and goats or pigs. In the priest's garden in Vilcabamba there is the peculiar fruit called sweet lemon, extremely insipid to eat, all skin and under-skin, like chewing on paper. But the people of the place think it has remarkable qualities. It is flat on top like a tangerine, a brilliant green, but with very little juice.

The present church in Vilcabamba is about 150 years old. The original one stood among the old trees of the early village. Few of the country churches are very old; most of them are rarely over a hundred years old, as the inhabitants like to pull them down and erect others as soon as anyone in the village acquires wealth. (The font and the old church records are always retained.) The churches seem to imitate the potlatch system of the North American Indian tribes, in this, a prestige economy, to show that the village was thriving. Even one person becoming rich in the village was enough. This occurred, too, in neighboring capitals of South America, such as Bogotá and Lima, where they pulled down the churches as some of the population became more and more wealthy, and built others in keeping with the new architecture. The result is that these capitals are not nearly so attractive as is Quito now. (Only because Quito was very poor as a capital have its original cathedrals and churches remained.)

The church at Vilcabamba is very high and airy, with enough room for the whole population. The colors inside are rather faded and very beautiful. The floor is tiled, and painted in very light colors, as is the ceiling. This made the whole very light even when the sun had gone. There are chairs for the congregation. Around the sides are processional crosses, images on the walls and several paintings. Very few of these are valuable or old, in any of the villages (unlike in Quito, where you can see many old masters on the walls of some of the bigger churches—the Cathedral and San Francisco Church date back to the sixteenth century). There is a font in the back of the church, similar to those found in England. The fonts are often much older than the existing church, as they were taken and retained from the older one. The most interesting item in the Vilcabamba church is a small altar dedicated to the grotto at Lourdes, with a small grotto made of stones. This was made about eighty years ago and has become quite famous since then.

Along the other side of the plaza in Vilcabamba are the larger houses of the town, some rather rural-looking government offices and a few shops that seemed to sell chiefly hats, some bottles of Pepsi-Cola of ancient vintage (probably homemade), biscuits (looking uncommonly like dog biscuits), pasta (looking like macaroni). There are also piles of tinned food. In fact they look very similar to the cheaper shops of Loja and elsewhere in Ecuador. In a few of them there are also some tables with plastic covers, and attendant flies, found the world over from Bangkok to Valparaiso in small local cafes; and here, as elsewhere, is the origination of many unusual types of dysentery found in the food. Strange to have cafes like these—dusty, airless and half dark—with all the beautiful mountains around and the excellent climate. It would have been more attractive to have had the chairs outside. On the benches along many of the verandahs sit cowboy types, complete with their six-shooters.

On the elaborate steps that run the length of the ecclesiastical plateau, there are usually people sitting and talking to their friends during the daytime. On Sundays they are the hub of the village. The main mass is at twelve o'clock, when people come from far and near to attend. Most of the service relies on the effort of the priest. The people partake very little apart from joining in the Kyrie eleison. The service takes about an hour, and then they pour out down the steps. At the base of the steps there is quite a gathering, people in little groups chatting to each other about the latest news, usually for at least two hours. Here and there are images, with lights, being carried by individual family groups who have been involved in a birth, a marriage or a death. Arrayed between the steps and the middle of the plaza are a row of stalls where a great variety of items are sold—from clothes to wooden trenchers. This is a kind of Sunday trading market for the produce of the village and the nearest town—bread, sugar, coffee, rice, pasta, beer. In Quito these venders come right into the portals of the cathedral—in spite of a huge painting at the entrance showing Christ clearing out the money-changers and merchants with a whip! The market lasts about two hours. Other people are content to gossip to their friends, and it looks very much like a country scene, with the three hundred or so people congregated on the steps and in the precincts of the church.

Gradually they disperse, taking a look as they go at the stores selling wares such as dried fish and meat. The meat stall is hidden from the mainstream of people—the stall holders seem very sheepish about it being there at all, because their stalls sell all parts of the animal, and the smell and look is often very disgusting. In San Pedro the people meet around the corner away from the main square, which they consider to be too public with the vehicles going through to Peru.

They have many committees in the village—the villagers love this kind of function. One of these committees was for the Reception of Cardiologists, but recently they had to change this to the Committee for the Reception of Tourist, for many are now coming. Any heart patient, from any part of the world, improves after a visit to the village. Certainly the few so far who have been there have, without exception, got better in two or three months, even though their lips and their fingers were black when they arrived in the valley, so serious was their condition.

The priests are interesting and dress in a singular fashion. The priest in Vilcabamba always wore a tammy but as soon as he went out he donned a very ancient and imposing pith helmet. Most of them wear a patched cassock with burn holes, covered with dirty marks and candle grease. The priest at Vilcabamba completed his ensemble with baseball boots and carried a stick like a shepherd's crook. Often they have several days' growth of beard on their faces; often, too, they look young for their ages. The priest at Vilcabamba was sixty-seven and had been there three years.

The priest of San Pedro was a little different. He was younger and often wore civilian dress, usually a brown suit and a tammy also. He had been the priest at Vilcabamba for three years. His name was Angel Soto and his place had been taken in Vilcabamba by Francisco Bravo (still the priest there); Angel Soto got rheumatism and that was the reason he left. This is more or less the only disease that can be claimed to be troublesome in Vilcabamba. The only sickness I experienced there was a slight twinge of rheumatism.

Very little work is done on the weekends; the men are occupied in drinking, and the women in gossiping. Drinking is indulged in by most only on weekends; the men often drink steadily, usually on Saturday night, until they are completely "out," but they are generally sober on Monday morning. There was less drunkenness in San Pedro than in Vilcabamba. The priest there always had a ready glass for the visitor, but seemed to set a good example over drunkenness. Many fights occurred in the villages during the weekend; I think it may have been because their lives had been so placid during the week.

Most of the drink taken is a fresh form of rum, drawn off when sugar juice is being boiled; the liquid from the first boiling is drawn off and left to stand for two or three days. It tastes like sweet water and looks like pale, milkless tea. However, this ferments inside the stomach in about one hour and one becomes intoxicated. In every direction men could be seen staggering about on weekends. There is another kind of alcohol made from fermented maize which tastes like Japanese *saki*—besides *chicha*, which was originally made partly by a community of women spitting into a common bowl. But, even when intoxicated, they always seemed polite to the stranger and would insist on shaking hands. The men smoked anything from one to forty cigarettes a day. These are made from tobacco grown in the gardens, wrapped in maize leaves in Vilcabamba, but in San Pedro in the best crude toilet paper.

Walks are taken at weekends and several of the young inhabitants make up a party and climb the mountains—much more enterprising than their town cousins, who stare at anyone in climbing boots as if they had come from another planet. I looked out at Mandango one day and saw a stream of people like so many multicolored ants, gradually meandering up the side of the mountain. The schools have holidays to make these expeditions, and often the people would sing as they went. I was delighted to see them, for I wanted to find the way up. I had hopes of climbing the mountains at a later date, when we were less busy in making out records of the people. It was interesting, too, to see the wild cattle and horses high up on the mountains, aiming for the remote scrub areas to avoid the invasion of humans that they could sense were coming. Only the observers down below could see this. These pilgrimages happen about four times a year. All the highest peaks, which are about 5,000 meters in height, are well marked with crosses that could just be seen from below, made and erected by past climbers; after a pilgrimage has been made, these are festooned with scarves and discarded clothing by the successful schoolboy explorers.

Clothes are very similar to those worn by agricultural workers in England, but more rugged and generally very patched. Villagers either go barefoot or wear homemade sandals, plaited, of grass or leather. Often the trousers are cut off short, leaving the brown and muscular calves bare. The men wear superb panamas. These are for sale at the best of the village stalls; they come in many varieties—the larger the weave the cheaper they are. Sometimes they have leather thongs around the brim. In San Pedro they went in more for wider straw hats or trilbies.

The women wear proper straw hats, often of the bright, varnished variety decorated with flowers that one used to see in Sunday schools. They look like poor English country women from the latter half of the nineteenth century, going out to do gleaning. They are a very pleasant sight, after the dull dresses and trilbies of the Quito Indians. The girls attempt to wear gay things but their life of drudgery often prevents them. Women are little admired in this region; on the whole they are regarded as objects, to be enjoyed when young, and for work when old. The women of San Pedro have broader faces and look much healthier than those of Vilcabamba.

A typical day in the life of one of these villages passes something like this. The first signs of the dawn are at about 6:10 A.M. each day. But at about 6:00 A.M. the whole of the valley is filled with the cock's clarion call, followed very quickly by the cry of the drongos—lovely birds, with large black long tails and hooked beaks. They have a repertoire of wonderful calls. Mingling with these is the braying of multitudes of donkeys. This is soon followed by the dogs' chorus; it starts by a little high-pitched yap of a puppy and includes, toward the end, the deep baying of hounds. In addition, in Vilcabamba, there is the grunting of the midget pigs, while in San Pedro there is the bleating of goats. No one seems inclined to get up before dawn and even then it is not a particularly hurried stirring. There being no lavatories, trips are made to the nearby fields, usually bringing in the eggs, maize or other items at the same time, for the first frugal repast of the day. This may consist of black coffee, followed either by a sweet kind of bread and the drinking egg—which is an uncooked egg broken into a glass—or by maize soup, made chiefly of maize cooked in water and including anything else that happens to be handy— herbs, perhaps pigs' fat or skin, and the gizzard of a chicken. These last are rather rare—more commonly it is an egg. They eat only about one ounce of meat a week. Cheese, which is not used up is eaten next day, or even several days later. With time, it developes a patina, and a deep yellowish hue beneath. Squares of pasta are also added by way of variety.

Nearly everyone has some function in the life of the community; all seem to go off into the fields, even those who live in the village. The land surrounding the village is parceled up into small holdings, and the *campesinos,* or peasants, rely on them for the food that is produced. The system of agriculture is a relic from the old colonial times, with its wooden, bullock-drawn plows and bullock carts. The rate of pay in the area is low, about ten sucres (fifty cents) per day. It varies according to the work. For the grinding of corn a little more is paid. Women are much used as labor in the harvesting of the coffee crops, which is very precise work. There are more women than men in the region: for example, in Vilcabamba, there are four hundred men and six hundred women.

Many of the centenarians also work on the land—José María Roa wades through ooze from which he makes adobe. Miguel Carpio, once a hunter, retired from this fifty years ago and is now a farmer. Walking up the steep slopes and through the thick mud increases the efficiency of their hearts—certainly an aid to health, and possibly to longevity. Others work in the village: Michaela

Quezada, who is 102, spins sheep's wool in front of her house in the village; Hermelinda Leon works in the bakery usually one or two days a week, and cultivates her garden for the remainder of the week.

Fruit is eaten throughout the day by those people in the fields. The climate is ideal for citrus fruits, and there are many other kinds of hedgerow fruits, such as mora (a cross between a raspberry and a blackberry), guava and naranjhuila; the last two are not very appetizing to the uninitiated, for it is difficult to come across a ripe fruit that is not plentifully supplied with maggots. At midday, coffee is drunk, often brought to the fields by the women of the farm.

The chief meal of the day is in the evening, taken about 5:00 P.M., allowing plenty of time before darkness comes about 6:15 P.M. This meal is made up of very small wild potatoes, yucca, cottage cheese, maize and a maize or bean gruel. Melons make up the dessert. The old probably only eat the gruel and the soft fruit. (In San Pedro, there is less fruit eaten and more milk and cheese.) They often eat corn cobs also, which are taken in a bag for lunch. They might munch some sugar cane too along the way. Popcorn and some meat might be put in the soup. Occasionally in the shops in Vilcabamba some dried fish, usually half bad can be bought; and yet in the rivers, especially the Quinara, very good fish can be found. But fishing is not a recreation of the people. As Vilcabamba and these other villages are some way from the sea some women get goiter through lack of iodine. Unfortunately for the village people's health, if they can get white bread, sugar, white rice and pasta, they add these to their diet.

The mountain people's diet is frugal; they never see white bread, and rice, sugar and pasta are delicacies. It is probably this lack of access to the more expensive foods that has helped them to live so long.

The countryman does not usually wear a hat, except a few of the very old, who wear Balaclava helmets. They have no real need for headgear, unless they are out in the hot sun, as they have such good heads of hair—especially in San Pedro.

Many of the children of the village, especially the girls, amuse themselves by playing games such as cat's cradle—surely a universal game! Most of the boys have a catapult, and no bird or animal is safe from these. It is used more in Vilcabamba than elsewhere. Another game they play is whipping wooden tops.

A hundred years ago there were large groves of fruit trees in these villages, as we see from the old site of Vilcabamba, where the lovely orange groves still remain. Even these may go soon for the land is suitable for growing sugar cane. In Vilcabamba, more than elsewhere, there are signs that there had been very large trees, probably eucalyptus; their stumps can still be seen. Originally many more herbs were grown—now, these can only be found in patches of waste ground where the soil is unsuitable for growing sugar cane. The mountains were probably also more clothed with large trees and there were fewer cattle in previous periods. Many more springs and water holes existed; often these have been spoiled by cattle using them, breaking down their edges until they have become almost ponds instead of clear, neat little shallow wells, as they were originally. The cattle are very prolific; the guayuna herb, which is thought to increase fertility, has spread everywhere. Much emphasis is laid on fertility—in fact the general feeling is that everything must be reproducing, their cattle and their women.

The arrival of sugar cane as the primary crop has led to the plowing up of many of the smaller fields and orchards in the vicinity of the village. The small mills where the sugar cane is processed are liable to start up at any time of the night, depending entirely on how much of the cane has been cut and piled up at the side of the mill. Both man and donkey, in the harvest seasons, work day and night; and many do piecework in order to feed or partially feed their large families. The donkey's life expectancy with this harsh life is not high; and most of them have some physical deformity. Most of the sugar is sold in brickettes and taken to the nearest large towns. A brick can be bought for about a sucre—that is, about 2 pence a kilo. I have seen none at San Pedro, where they have no fields of sugar cane.

In some of the small fields, owned by the poorest of farmers, wooden plows drawn by large oxen are still in use. These are yoked, so that most of the strain is taken by the head and neck. Besides making the beasts strain at an awkward angle, much energy is lost in this way. There are also wooden contraptions for dehusking the corn, and other, simple machines for collecting the plant juices and for pressing tobacco leaves. These are often crude. Farmers make good use of tree logs, cutting out a rectangular hollow in them, and using a wooden dumper. They often crush the corn cobs in them. Many people make full use of their back garden to grow maize and tobacco. Tobacco is put on a line in front of the house to dry, after it has been crushed in the machine. In Vilcabamba, coffee beans are put out in the road to dry on mats; they are brought in again in the evening so that the dew will not spoil them. As there is so little traffic they are quite safe there.

The bread of Vilcabamba is famous (and very sweet). The special kind of oven that they use for baking it is made of mud or clay and looks very similar to an igloo. The only large industries in the region are converting sugar juice into blocks of candy, manufacturing rum and making bread. When the women decide to have a baking day, they announce this to all and sundry by hanging out a white cloth on the largest tree near their house, so that people can come and buy their bread and cakes.

There is very little wildlife on the sierras, as the extreme poverty that most of the people live in makes them hunt for all possible—and some impossible—food, even the porcupine and the armadillo. Only those creatures which have a very strong capacity for survival, or those too cunning or repulsive for the hunters to kill, manage to survive, such as raccoonlike animals and wolves. It is an interesting example of what happens to the creatures in a land where there are no protective conservation methods.

The people do not sing as they work in the fields, but when they relax they sing to the accompaniment of a guitar. Most of their songs are ballads about local heroes and the sexual prowess of those heroes; and they will serenade girls at night. Once or twice, I heard a burst of song and a guitar, at two or three in the morning, at a house where one of the prettiest girls lived. There are also pan pipes, which have a melancholy sound: the men only seem to play them if they have been crossed in love. They can be bought for about five sucres in the towns of that region, but most of them are made by the player, of several reed or young bamboo pipes strung together. Their beautiful but sad music can be heard from a great distance.

There are very few influences of the twentieth century outside the villages themselves. There are no airplanes flying overhead; few if any small holders own transistor radios; there is no smoke in the air—it is crystal clear. A hundred years ago there were probably more clothes of the home-spun variety, as all the women did their family's weaving. Today this is left increasingly to the old. One can still see women walking along the country lanes, spinning as they go, driving their herds about. They occasionally wet the wool that they are spinning so that it evolves into a thread. Many of the very old women are seamstresses until the end of their days, this being more commonly seen in the San Pedro community than in the others. Cotton is used for clothing more in San Pedro than elsewhere. As soon as the sewing machine comes, many will give up the art of spinning as it is known today.

The daily routine of the mountain people follows that of the sun even more closely than that of the villagers. People use their houses only for storing things and for resting. Their beds are large, often made of bamboo, with bamboo struts as the only springs. At the end of the bed they keep a bundle of clothes, all that they possess. Small hens like bantams, perched on their brown eggs, sit on top of the verandahs that surround the houses. Most of the houses are situated on patches hollowed out of the hillside and generally there is a bamboo fence around the immediate vicinity of the house. Beyond this is a small meadow for the animals, fenced to keep them out of the small, unfenced fields with their crops.

What is a typical day in the life of a centenarian? After all, these are the people who made this spot so particularly interesting for us. The life of the centenarians in the village is similar to that found in most rural villages in South America. Village life is likely to be less interesting for them than life on the mountain small holdings where most of them live (unless they are unable to manage for themselves). There is much less desire for conformity in the small holdings, and far less encroachment of the "plastic culture." Life in the little valleys, where the sun streams down each day, is marvelously invigorating and has much simple beauty.

Long before the dawn the call of the cock, from a hundred little farms or more, would prepare the morning. The fox's bark, hunting waterfowl by some hidden stream, echoes from crag to crag. This wakes Gabriel, a centenarian, from his bed—and the scratching of a pig against the hut makes him more aware of his surroundings! Then the two-inch stump of candle, perched on a stalagmite of wax (not an inch of the basic bottle showing through) is lit.

By his bed the centenarian mutters a prayer to his Lord and Maker, stirs his wife Rosa from her side of the bed, and in the dim light of the candle she gropes for some of her clothes that have a permanent home at the end of the crude wooden bed. The centenarian gropes for a basket at the side of a pile of hoes in one corner and a knife from one of the rafters, and creaks open the roughhewn door of the hut; and then to the verandah outside. Here he is greeted by the serenade of many birds. The sky is now streaked with red—for dawn comes quickly to the valley, being so close to the Equator.

Most of the houses are small and have about five people living there: a centenarian, his wife, one of his daughters, a granddaughter, possibly a great-granddaughter, and this would make up the household. The rest of the family would be found on a small holding next door, or possibly even a mile away.

From the back of the little house there stretches a path, forever it seems, leading upward through the stunted trees and a small patch of sugar cane—and leads eventually to the little patchy maize fields that are scattered over certain sections of the mountainside. Our centenarian takes this path as the sun peeps over Warango ridge; many small birds fly up as he passes along, basket in hand. The path is still damp from the heavy dew or from the light showers that fall (but only at night). Up he climbs as if it were to meet the sun. Somewhere down below him his wife is also starting out in a search for eggs from the bantams that lay in the surrounding shrub. The path he follows now would be almost impossible for a European, as it leads around the edge of a secluded canyon; soon this is negotiated and he is in his little field which has been developed from the rocky soil that surrounds it. Walls of stone taken from its surface surround it—this work was

done by his forefathers. There are about three hundred head of
corn in this field; as he fills his basket with some, the view below is
smudged with the smoke of one hundred farms, and within half
an hour he is back at the house.

His daughter and granddaughter have now emerged from their
little rooms and are on the verandah waiting for the first meal of
the day to begin. Stools are placed in front of the shaped tree
trunks that act as benches on the verandah and on these are
placed an assortment of plates for the flat cake of white cheese,
lightly boiled eggs, homemade brown bread, boiled beans and
now the lightly boiled corn cobs. These are eaten heartily and
washed down with spring water. Down at the village in the valley
there are flies everywhere; not so around these huts in the mountains—there is not a fly to be seen anywhere, and no other harmful
insects for that matter; only myriads of butterflies, around the
house and along the way.

When their repast is over the youngest, the granddaughter,
leaves first for the village. Her grandmother, Rosa, who is now
close to a hundred, then wanders off to the nearby scrub to search
for wood for the oven, for today it is baking day. The oven is first
packed with brushwood and then set alight. After two hours all
the ash is scraped out with a special tool and the dough that has
been prepared in the meantime is placed, with the aid of a long,
flat spadelike instrument, on the still simmering floor. The door is
shut, and not opened again for another two hours. The white flag
is then hoisted to let everyone know where bread can soon be obtained. The centenarian's wife has been doing this job since her
early teens and feels it no hardship. She, like Michaela Quesada,
who is now nearly 105, hopes to be carrying on this work for several more years. When she is not doing this task she accompanies
her husband to the field, she carrying the dinner, her husband carrying their two hoes, and there they work side by side. They continue in such a manner for long hours although they can no longer
do the hard work of breaking up new ground and carrying the
stones off it. This work would be left to the men twenty or thirty
years younger, and continued up to their late eighties. When the
nineties are reached they begin to look for the lighter tasks, but
the work is as regular, day in, day out, as before.

Today, after the baking is over and the loaves have been made, Rosa will go to the field to meet her husband when the sun is high; for today, with several others, they will go to visit the shrine of Petridos—the spring that gushes out of a sheer rock face high above the village, part of the Mandango mountain.

For her lunch she eats a couple of corn cobs and for her husband she places three, still warm from the cooking pot, in a cloth. She then treads the path made so familiar from many years of toil. It seems hard and dry now for it is the hottest part of the day, but she negotiates a place where the path has given way, and does not look down at the hundred-foot drop below. She finds her husband resting in the shade of an old wild orange tree which still has some blossom on it, and also some masses of fruit. She tumbles out the corn cobs onto the grassy verge and, while her husband is munching away, she plucks the ripest of the fruit for their dessert. Not lingering for more than a few minutes after the meal is over, they start on their way to the shrine, which is much higher up on the mountain. Already streaks of color can be seen as little crocodiles of people ahead zigzag up the mountainside.

They pass a farm here and there, and greet the people with a wave, pausing for a few moments to allow them to leave their work and join the band with bottles and containers to bring down some of the precious water. One farmer, though very old, is repairing a fence to prevent his cows trampling on a neighbor's crops. The younger brother of our farmer, Gabriel, getting on for 120, will leave the task that he has been doing for most of the morning, that of treading the ooze that will be made into adobe bricks when baked in the sun, an activity very beneficial for the circulation. He goes to wash his legs in the nearby trickle and does not bother to roll down his trousers or put on his sandals, but joins the throng just as he is.

The groups arrive, singing, at the holy well. Some are resting on the grassy banks before entering the wood where the spring is, others are just entering. When they arrive at the spring they kneel as if in prayer, or at the altar for communion, and then either drink a deep draught or collect some of the water in one of the utensils that they have brought along—some do both, silent from their song only while they drink the crystal waters. In spite of so many trampling feet the spring is still clean, unlike the other holy springs farther down in the valley which are also popular with various kinds of domestic animals.

The day has not finished for them yet. They return home for another, and final, meal—not too late for it is always "home before dark." When the meal is over the younger members of the family who have prepared it will clear away; Gabriel will sit on the verandah, repair and sharpen his tools or mend his sandals, perhaps even make another stool or two. Rosa also will sit on the verandah with the ever-changing sun making her hair glisten, the mountains now green, now purple, beyond. But she is not idle, for we find that she is neatly sewing or embroidering, often in many colors, with no sign of strain in her eyes.

Sometimes, when they are reaching the end of their days, they will complain to the younger members of the family that they can no longer see the other side of the valley quite so clearly. Sometimes, too, they will complain that the birds do not sing quite so well as when they ran about the valleys as boys!

It is then time for bed. It is early, but they sleep with the sun— up at 5:30 A.M. and to bed at 7:30 P.M.

10

The Authenticity
of the Ecuadoran
Centenarians

There are reports from time to time in the newspapers of people living to be great ages. Alas, in these days they are usually to be found in old people's homes. They are authentic in England, which has a superb system of checking—the Public Records Office. At the time of writing, Britian's oldest woman, Miss Alice Stevenson, has died at the age of 112, in an old people's home in Sutton, Surrey. We can vouch for the authenticity of her age with ease because of this record system. This remarkable old lady died just after her birthday, on 10 July 1973, though not through a surfeit of celebrating! This is an interesting psychological point, for the majority of the very ancient die like this. It is as if they are motivated by something to live for and to look forward to, for example their birthday celebration, and the excitement and interest this arouses in their often rather dull routine. Alice Stevenson was deaf and almost blind—very different from the people whom we find in Ecuador.

Males generally remain alive longer than females in those reaching ages above 105, especially if they can avoid prostate gland trouble. Most of the oldest ladies are spinsters. These people have a strong constitution, maintaining a good metabolism.

Yet some live a vegetable existence toward the end, and this is a state that everyone wishes to avoid. Man is forever seeking immortality in some form or another, and to live to a lucid hundred years is one of them. It is worth investigating to see if there is anything in our environment that could help greater active longevity.

There are many legends and tales about long life. There is the soma plant of the Indian continent, which is fully described in the *Kama Sutra*—but no one seems to be able to obtain specimens. One of this plant's remarkable properties is said to be to rejuvenate people. The juice is extracted from the bulb and the "cure" takes seven weeks. To live entirely on grapes is also said to aid longevity. Certainly the Caucasian centenarians drink a great deal of wine.

Then there are the Buddhist priests who try the mystical way, and who are known by the local inhabitants to occupy a particular cave for seventy years—yet still seem to look young at the end of their existence. Doubters would say that it was obvious that they move caves, and thus different monks re-emerge. An interesting book on this subject is by Thoms; he was the chief of the doubters, and refutes the story of "Old Parr" and the other remarkable examples of longevity. "Old Parr" is reputed to have been the oldest man to have lived in the Western world. He lived in South Wales in the eighteenth and nineteenth centuries. But Thoms makes much of the fact that it was a very common practice to hand down names, and how the 154 years that he is considered to have reached are the combined ages of father and son rolled into one.

Isolated examples of people living to very great ages are interesting as individual cases—but they hold no key to our search. We want to find *groups* of people who have a high percentage of centenarians in their midst. Genetic factors may play a part, but the interest of these groups in Ecuador is that the likelihood is much greater that here environmental factors are also responsible. Though genetics can be a base, we must have the bricks and mortar—the environment.

In Ecuador, there is a very high percentage of aged people in some of the communities. For example, in San Pedro there are 88 people above the age of 80 in a community of 760 people. The repetition of family and Christian names is very unlikely to be a confusing factor in South America, for besides the name of the father, children retain the surname of the mother and they nearly always have two Christian names. There is also often an Indian element, so that some of them may have Indian names as well. It is very rare to have any repetition, therefore, in such a string of names.

If we followed the course of any one of the individual centenarians with regard to habits, diet etc., this would be no criterion or blueprint for a general theory of how to live longer. But if we follow up in detail the diet of an isolated group of centenarians, then the information obtained might be more significant. Unfortunately, there is as yet no *physical* way of detecting the age of a person. There often may be no authentic record of the beginning of their lives, such as baptismal certificates which bring us within six months of their actual ages. The Ecuadorans *do* have such certificates. Much more reliance has to be placed on hearsay military records and passports in the case of the Russians and people living in Moslem countries. This makes the task much more difficult and unreliable. We think of people as old from the age of eighty upward, but those of uncertain old age are useful only as cross-checks with age-known specimens, and for comparisons in regard to diet etc.

In our search for the reasons for longevity we must first of all look at aging in people who are age-known specimens. When we have facts on these, such as diet, altitude, herbs, trace elements in their environment, we can see if we can find similarities among the unverified old of the rest of the world. At present we cannot often seek the help of the medical profession in these studies, as many of them feel that the study of herbs and trace elements would make them little better than witch doctors!

Baptismal certificates of people still living date back to April 1847 (Francisco Camacho of Sacapalca) and others recently dead to 1845. (The previous world record is 113 years.) There is no reason to suppose that these are not authentic. Again, there are certificates for people of lesser ages in the region—120 years or so of age (Rosauia Cango and David Castillo Calderon of La Chota). Then we find death certificates of four people who lived to 150 years of age and died in the 1920s and 1930s in Cangonama, Cariamanga, Catacotcha and San Pedro, where the records go back to the early eighteenth century. I can think of no reason why the Jesuits should falsify these documents: they would not want to attract visitors to the area, for this was where the Peruvian bark (or quinine tree) was to be found. The Jesuits got a huge levy from this, as they controlled its exports (until an Englishman smuggled some seeds out of the country), and it was the only thing that relieved the almost universally found malarial fevers for many years.

These people of South America are the nearest to perfect samples to study in depth. Furthermore, they are found where there are few political problems (except for the fact that it is a frontier area), which is not the case with the Russians and the regions of Pakistan and China where the Hunzas are found. To complete this task of study and research may take a few years; however, we hope by that time the world will be in a better position than today to accept and digest the knowledge of mankind gained in these open-air laboratories.

A parallel study should also be made of the animals in the valleys, to see what secrets they might have to give. We may find the reaching of a great age in humans has much to do with living, by our standards, a half-starved existence. (Recently at Cambridge University some studies were carried out upon rats, and it was found that if these were kept in a half-starved state, they lived a third as long again as the well-fed rats. Recently, also at Cambridge, A. N. Howard of Downing College fed a hundred rats on butter for only fifty days, and they all died of heart attacks.) These Ecuadoran people seem to avoid getting the killing diseases of the heart and cancer. Why? Yet when they are infants about 40 per cent die before they reach their fourth year from the usual epidemics and viruses—the civil registers tell us this. But in the process of growing up they become immune to many diseases and after their teens they seem very hardy physically.

In our studies of these villages, we found the padres, the village priests, reliable in every way, and what they told us we found, on checking, to be accurate. If someone came in with a report that a man was 116, the priests would check in the registers, showing them to us also. If the report was wrong, they would tell us and give the correct age. These men could not have been better guardians of the books; they would not let them out of their sight, though we were allowed to photograph and handle them as much as we liked. But the books could not leave the church premises. The earlier were made of parchment, with a skin covering. The earliest books of San Pedro and Gonzanamá were like this, and in the case of Gonzanamá they date back to 1655. After 1750, they were still leather-bound but the pages were of paper (on which were often authentic blots). These are still highly legible, for whoever did the clerking made sure that they were well written, often beautifully so. Many of these books are, in fact, in a better condition than those to be found in our own church safes. The climate of the sierra, at least where the centenarians are found, is very dry (perhaps this may contribute to their longevity), and this has helped to preserve the books.

In the majority of cases, the registers can be read very clearly. Sometimes the age is in numerals, but more often it is expressed in words. The registers come in two forms. Those that belong to the church give all the details one would expect: the child's legitimacy and parents. The second belong to the state, the civil registers. These are entirely secular, and are housed in a separate office in the village—usually that of the *teniente político* agent. Most of these go back to 1900 when such features of civil administration got under way. They are quite intriguing as they go into details of when a person died, what he died of—gripes (flu) and measles, etc.—and we see here the evidence of the terrible infant mortality of the region, and also what are the common ailments. Used together, they give a full picture.

What these certificates did show was that these people living to great ages were no flash in the pan. The region had, as far back as the records went, showed the same pattern.

Some villages did not possess their old registers, and one had to go elsewhere for them. Sometimes the child would be registered in the chief town of the district and not at the village where he was born and this required some hunting. Another difficulty was the number of illegitimate births, which might or might not have been put in—according to the whim of the individual priest.

The very early records of Vilcabamba were at Malacatos—about an hour's jeep ride from Vilcabamba.

In some instances, we met people who carried around a copy of their own birth certificates, but for the most part these were quite unreadable, and the owners were often only in their eighties.

While we were checking the documents, word would get around that the foreigners were there, and people of all ages would come to the priest's office. The little boys would arrive first, in anticipation of having their photos taken along with the "exhibits." The priest and an experienced "disperser" would be in attendance to try to get rid of them. Our photographer would try bribery, by making a flash that they enjoyed as much as any firework display. Soon the very old would arrive, and expect to be asked questions. When the crowd outside became too large, we would take pictures of the registers inside. On one occasion the church bell tolled to let them know what was happening in their village, the result being that the old came in from far and near; some continued to come hours after the bell had ceased to toll.

The whole of Ecuador has such registers, and these are an excellent way of noting very quickly if there is anything unusual in a village, whether centenarians, or the opposite (as is seen more often in some of the villages in Peru, where the people age rapidly and die comparatively young). But usually a place with some unique quality is well known locally. We generally heard from the old people themselves where they were born, and they would tell us that there were others of a great age to be found there also. Or one of the priests would inform us, and we would go along on the appointed day to take a look at the registers. This was our method of approach for locating the centenarians, once we had started to study the diets of the region.

On my return to England after the first visit, my colleagues, hearing about these centenarians, asked whether there was any documentary evidence (remembering the Caucasians). I made a point of having plenty of photographic evidence of living people, certificates of birth, baptism and death, in order to show the authentication of their ages.

With the majority of the centenarians, we investigated their relatives and found their sons and grandsons to be elderly or middle-aged. For instance, the grandson of Miguel Carpio was 49. Miguel Carpio himself was very lucid, and told of events such as invasions and wars—particularly the Peruvian one of 1894, in which he took part, and also the second one in 1912. His mind was clear over these events. He had a nephew of 94 who told us much about his famous uncle. Then there were three old women of the village, including Michaela Quesada Mendieta (104) who told us how they remembered Miguel as a young man when they were small girls. Each interview was held separately, so they could not prompt each other. This is remarkable for it shows that they had retained their memories, just as had Miguel Carpio himself. Usually in the West, people begin to lose their memory soon after deafness, which generally comes first. Most of us in old age have a much more sluggish blood supply to the brain than when we are younger and more active, mainly because we have less blood and the arteries on the side of the head atrophy; but these old people in Ecuador have plenty of blood flowing to their brains.

We found that we could talk to the people of Palmyra to get information on people of Vilcabamba, for there was much communication between the two places. From the top of mounts Mandango or Warango, both villages could be seen at the same time, lying in their valleys. We also gained much information from the children and other relatives of the centenarians when we were carrying out the medical examinations, and using questionnaires on them. Their answers all tallied, and they gave the ages of the centenarians correctly.

Thus we have been entirely satisfied that the ages of these centenarians are authentic. The most vital evidence was the baptismal certificates, but we always crossed and double-checked from the centenarians' own accounts, that of their friends and relatives, and other villagers, as well as connecting the dates of various events. This authenticity has given a special significance to this study of the Ecuadoran centenarians; authenticity has been much less easy to establish among the Abkhasians in Russia and the Hunzas on the Chinese/Pakistan border.

11

The Attitude of the Communities to the Centenarians

We wanted to compare the treatment of and attitude toward the centenarians and the other old people in the Andes with that of modern Western society.

The very old were more than tolerated; the rest of the community accepted them very fully, knowing that one day they, too, would be old. They were seen as capable of work, and having knowledge and wisdom, due to their years. In no instances that we saw were they living separate lives from the rest of the community.

The centenarians on the mountain small holdings never lived alone either. As mentioned earlier, about five people lived in each house, one or two middle-aged daughters and one or two teen-age granddaughters or great-granddaughters. Rarely did we see babies in these households. The overflow of the families would live in a house nearby. It was part of the social structure never to have very large houses, perhaps because of the danger of earthquakes. The old would pass on the crafts and arts they had learned, such as spinning and weaving.

Strangely, though great care and concern was shown among different members of a family, there was not a great deal of visiting or calling on each other. They did not seem particularly close to their children, or vice versa. They would meet each other regularly after church on Sunday mornings, but otherwise meetings were not frequent.

All the centenarians that we saw, except those who were in the heart of the villages, were living a useful life, keeping themselves and even others going. Perhaps their jobs were not always the heavier ones—breaking up new ground before planting the maize, or husking the rice (though some did do very heavy work, making adobe etc.)—but they had their own jobs of work in the community, such as getting the wood, getting up in the morning with the youngest children and putting them to bed, baking the local bread. When we visited Gabriel Sánchez, we had to await his arrival from the maize field, his great-granddaughter of eleven going to call him in from the field. We saw the tools that he brought back: one was a metal crowbar, used not only for fencing but for breaking up the earth. In his case he was taking his place in the front line with the young men! About 50 per cent of the male population of forty in our Western society could not use one of these effectively!

These people retain their youth in many ways. From their walk you would not think that they were very old. In order to get to Gabriel Sánchez's building it was necessary to cross a river by way of a pole and a wire. We all found this quite difficult, and on our return by the same route were planning to take some pictures of the hazard when, along the path on the other side, came a figure with a bundle of bamboo poles. These were about ten feet long, very awkward and heavy, for they had just been cut. Without hesitation, and hardly touching the wire, an old man set foot on the pole and almost ran across. When he got to our side I went up to him for a chat and he did not put the bundle down until asked to do so by the Ecuadoran doctor with us. He squatted down beside us on the bank. He was very lean and seemed all beard (part brown and part black with only a small amount of gray). His eyes had the same merry twinkle that I had seen in Miguel Carpio's and many other centenarians in the valleys. He was very lean and really looked like a man of the woods. We asked him his age, and he was ninety-five. This we checked with the priest's records and we found that Yuan Patrillo, who was still carrying these poles without much trouble, was indeed ninety-five.

He evidently owned some of the land near the river for he went back after depositing his load, and fetched some more while we were resting. On our way back, the last sight that we had of him was trying to pull a most reluctant cow by a halter into a daisy-covered meadow. There was something very boyish about him: as if he were a boy masquerading as an old man in a school play. One got the rather eerie feeling that he was going to disappear into the mountainside. All his faculties seemed to be present. We did not find this so much with the old women, but they developed a majesty in their old age—something like Queen Victoria!

Many people would find the lives they lead too hard by Western European standards—day in and day out the same monotonous grind, the same monotonous diet—climbing the steep path half a mile up the mountain in the morning sunshine, in order to get the breakfast of maize.

Their reactions to us wanting to study them were helpful; they were not at all upset by the battery of cameras they had to face. Even when photographs of their mouths were being taken (which must have been very trying) they co-operated, as long as they understood what we were doing. They did not give up at the end of the day; we did. The most friendly of all the villages that we visited was San Pedro de la Bendita. Such is the respect for the old here that even when they were infirm or became too old to look after themselves, the people would see that they were not neglected in any way. Only in Nambacola was there some sign of neglect, but this was because many people there were on the threshold of starvation themselves.

For some reason some of the old would sometimes try to reduce their ages, as if they were ashamed to admit that they were over seventy—less from vanity than not wishing to tempt fate. This was especially so of the women of San Pedro, and if one of them said that she was forty (when it was obvious that she was older) it would be a man who would go and check and tell us her real age. Such reluctance to reveal her age was probably because a woman did not wish to be termed a witch. It was unusual, as mostly the very old were proud of their age.

Clearly, this more positive attitude to the old, where they are not only included into life in the community, but their work and their wisdom are taken seriously by the younger people, is very different from our Western attitudes, where to be old is often thought to be synonymous with being useless. Though it is not a measurable factor, the psychological result of this positive view must undoubtedly affect the energies and optimism of the old people themselves and increase their wish to continue living—and this wish is known to be an important factor in the maintenance of a healthy and long life.

12

A Comparative Study
of the Centenarians
of Ecuador, Abkhasia
and the Hunzucuts

It is important here to take a look at some of the other communities renowned for their centenarians, and to compare them with the centenarians of Ecuador. Two groups are particularly interesting in this respect. One is the Abkhasians, to be found on the eastern shores of the Black Sea in the Caucasus mountains. The other group, the Hunzas, are divided geographically by a purely political division; part of this group is to be found in Pakistan and part in Sinkiang in China. They are extremely difficult to contact these days—again entirely for political reasons. In recent years a few British Council teachers have been there, but this was before Pakistan left the Commonwealth.

Only a few Western anthropologists and journalists have managed to reach the Abkhasians, who live in a rather rugged area, in many ways similar to that found in southern Ecuador. It is a region of hard land, and the Abkhasians term it "God's afterthought." But, like the setting of the Andean villages, it is beautiful. The Abkhasians, nearly all Muslims, have been there for at least a thousand years. There are now about 150,000 Abkhasians, and about 2,000 of these are reputed to be centenarians. About a quarter of the population of the Abkhasian republic is pure-

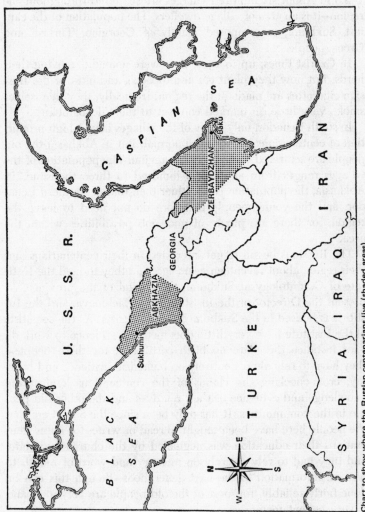

Chart to show where the Russian centenarians live (shaded areas).

blooded Abkhasian. The area is part of the Soviet Socialist Republic of Georgia, which itself is one of the republics that form the U.S.S.R. About six hundred villages are scattered throughout the region—it is an area of village dwellers. The population of the capital, Sukhumi, is composed mainly of Georgian, Turkish and Greek people.

In Czarist times, up to 1918, they were nomadic, moving their herds. But now they plant tea and tobacco, and most of the Russian cigarettes are made in the region. Ironically, they themselves smoke very little, in marked contrast to the Vilcabambans.

In south Ecuador, only a few of the villages have a high proportion of centenarians; the rest are normal. But in Abkhasia the old people are scattered throughout the region. The population of the villages ranges from about two hundred to three thousand. In Abkhasia, the population is wealthier than that of southern Ecuador, and the young people therefore do not need to leave the region, for there are plenty of good job possibilities within the area.

The Russians began to get interested in their centenarians and their region about seventeen years ago, and they formed the Institute of Gerontology at Sukhumi, the capital of the province. At present the Director of the Institute is Dr. Sichinava, and the Institute is housed in the Sukhumi Medical Center. As the scientists at the Institute have very little documentary evidence to work on —for instance there are no birth certificates for these people— they have to rely almost entirely on biological evidence and hearsay, cross-checking the claims of the centenarians against the knowledge and evidence of their relatives and the other old people in the communities. It has only been since the Soviet era that the people here have been taught to read or write; for many generations their education was neglected by the church and state, and they had to rely entirely on memory and word of mouth to pass on information to the next generations—though this can be done fairly reliably, for most of the old people are very alert and have excellent memories.

Even after death, and after studying the bones, we cannot tell the age of a deceased person exactly—only to within a few years. However the Russians, in spite of having no documentary evidence concerning their centenarians, are forging ahead with their research, and are in many ways far in advance of the rest of the world. If they had the wealth of authentic material that is available in Ecuador, they would by now have started a big research center in Loja.

A map of the Soviet Union will show that the Abkhasians live on the foothills of mountains close to the Black Sea. Most of the centenarians in the world have been found in the foothills or valleys of mountainous regions. It would be interesting to study more areas, such as Tibet.

To illustrate the life of an Abkhasian centenarian, I will take one or two examples. Among the Abkhasians the oldest inhabitant, until his death in 1973, was 168-year-old Shirali Mislimov, who lived in the village of Barzavu. One of his brothers died at the age of 134 and another younger brother of 106 also lived in the village. His father lived to be 120 and his mother 110. The village of Barzavu is high up in the mountains of Azerbaijan, not far from the Russo-Iranian border, and is in a setting very similar to Vilcabamba. Shirali Mislimov is believed to have left his village only twice in his lifetime: once to collect his first bride Leili, and once, recently, to visit Baku, the capital of the province. He was the son of a nomadic cattle herder, and could still remember in detail raids on the village from across the Iranian border, raids going back 150 years! He looked exceedingly smart right up to his death, and had a sharpness of mind that is also found in the Vilcabamban centenarians—a sharpness that seems to come rather than go with age! The similarities with the Ecuadorans do not stop there, for he had the same large ears and huge beaked nose. This may be due to an adaptive mechanism, fitting for survival purposes, where the lungs have to receive cold mountain air, which can be warmed in the well-developed nasal passages before it reaches the lungs. This type of nose is found on all mountain people and it shows a mountain origin. Shirali, like the majority of old people from his region, had no schooling. He was a shepherd until his "tribe" began to settle, and then he had to learn to farm. He was about the same height as the average Vilcabamban, that is about five feet six inches and, like them, very lean.

Two previous wives had died, including Leili, and at his death he was living with his third wife, a relative youngster of 107, whom he had married when he was 110! He claimed to have had very fulfilling marriages with the other two wives, saying that that was why he wanted another wife when widowed for the second time. Though a Muslim, he never had more than one wife at a time, possibly for economic reasons. His widow says that he was always very calm and good-tempered. From his three marriages, Shirali had twenty-three children, nine sons and fourteen daughters. Two daughters by his third wife are still living. As remarked earlier, very few of the people in the area move away. As a result, about 160 of his descendants live in the vicinity of Barzavu. His eldest great-granddaughter was seven when he died. He did not like town life, although he appeared to enjoy being somewhat of a celebrity.

Shirali kept all his faculties, right up to the time of his death. One eye was a little weak, but this had nothing to do with old age —it resulted from being hit in the eye by a stone when he was a boy. However, he only had two, very long, teeth in the front. This was a similarity he shared, unlike most Russian centenarians, with the Ecuadorans. In most cases the Abkhasians seem to have very good teeth. He had plenty of gray hair, a large gray beard— generally a grayer look than the centenarians of Ecuador. The centenarians of the Andes often have dark hair until well into their nineties, but both peoples have one thing in common: they rarely go bald. And both look much younger than their years.

Shirali quite probably had more money than such Vilcabambans as Miguel Carpio (123), Gabriel Sánchez (120) or Francisco Comacho (128), his counterparts in Ecuador, probably because his native region was more prosperous economically than that of his Ecuadoran peers. He certainly wore more fashionable clothes.

Shirali and his wife lived in the house of their forty-five-year-old married daughter. The house is similar to those in the sierra of Ecuador, complete with a verandah for leisurely gossips, reminiscences and meditations. Inside, it is not so bare as the Ecuadoran homes—the wooden floors are covered with woolen rugs. The houses are usually surrounded by a large garden, supplying the family with all the fruit and vegetables they need, apricots growing in particular abundance. The family, like the Ecuadorans, own cows, some sheep and poultry. Shirali's routine seldom changed throughout the years. He said his prayers at sunrise, like any good Muslim, and then went back to bed until seven or eight o'clock. After a short walk around the village he had his first repast of the day, which consisted of soured milk, mild sheep's cheese, freshly baked bread and tea. He then pottered around the garden, repairing the fences, sawing logs and looking after the animals. Like his South American peers, Shirali, too, kept in close contact with the farming community, especially with the farm where he had worked.

Right until the end of his life he had an excellent appetite, and rarely overate. He had three meals a day: the main midday meal was made up of rice soup, plenty of fresh vegetables, a milk dish, and, about once a week, some chicken or mutton. The evening meal was the same as breakfast. This diet is similar to that of the highlanders of Ecuador, except that the latter hardly ever eat meat. He, too, went to bed at sunset, and had a lot of sleep. But, in contrast to the Ecuadorans, he never drank strong drink or smoked. Despite his age he observed all the fasts laid down in the Koran.

He never went to see a doctor but as the years went by they became more and more interested in his health and welfare, checking up regularly on his state. They said that until quite shortly before his death his blood pressure and general health were more appropriate to a man of sixty. He himself attributed his age to his peaceful life—similar to the view of the Ecuadoran centenarians—the pure mountain air and the water from the mountain streams. He walked a good deal, and, on his regular visits to the gerontological center, covered the twelve miles there and back on foot, only occasionally with the help of a donkey.

Unlike the Ecuadorans, he had enough money to be hospitable and, like any good Muslim, always had a place for a visitor at his table. Of all company, he liked best that of young people. Carpio and Sánchez at Vilcabamba felt the same; they would bloom as soon as there were young people present—especially young girls! Shirali's best friend, Makmud Eivasov, died at the age of 153, about nine years ago. It was a severe blow to the old man, and his relatives say that he was never the same again. No longer could he talk about the old days to his friend.

Psychological self-doubt, which often comes with aging in Western communities, does not come with either of these groups. As a man's, or woman's, age increases so does his or her stature in the eyes of the community. An article in *The Sunday Times* in April 1966 gave an account of how a man of 123 sent his son of 50 into the fields to bring the horse in for harvesting. In about half an hour the son appeared, crestfallen, saying that the horse had given him the slip. Full of indignation the father stalked off and brought back the subdued horse. Not for him any doubts about his ability to do such a thing! It should be added that Abkhasian society, as southern Ecuadoran society, is patriarchal and patrilineal (importance and descent being invested in and through the father's family), the males being very powerful and the dominant members of the community.

Like the child, the old have a desire for security, and this is often found in the extended family. Among a kinship that may number several hundred, the old feel safe in the cocoon of relationships, and this may well be a factor in prolonging their lives. The high survival rate of the very old is also found in communities that value highly the continuity of their traditions; in such communities the old are indispensable in their transmission of wisdom and tales. Among the Abkhasians, the elders preside at important ceremonial occasions, they act as mediators in disputes, their words are respected to a high degree, their knowledge of farming is sought. They feel needed—and they are. The women also have a place in the community, for they teach the young girls weaving, sewing, knitting and cooking and many other arts that are vested in them. In Ecuador, the relationship of the old to the rest of the community is very similar.

Most of the Abkhasians work regularly almost to the end of their days, although not as hard as the Ecuadorans; again, this is probably for economic reasons. They still have good eyesight and their posture is unusually erect, both traits they have in common with the Ecuadorans. The Abkhasians swim a great deal in the mountain streams, unlike the old men of Ecuador. In Ecuador beards are worn, but the Abkhasians have a fondness for enor-

mous mustaches which give them an air of swashbuckling romanticism. In build they are very slim, and there is a saying that when
a man is lying on his side a dog should be able to pass between
him and the ground—such is the feeling about waists. The women
have a profusion of dark hair, but fair complexions.

Sula Benet, professor of anthropology at Hunter College in
New York City, tells us that in the village of Dzhgerda there were
71 men and 110 women between the ages of 81 and 90, and 19
people over 91—in other words, 15 per cent of the village population of 1,200. In 1954, the most recent date for which over-all
figures are available, 2.58 per cent of the Abkhasians were over 90.
The over-all figure for the Soviet Union is 0.1 per cent and the
figure for the U.S.A. is 0.4 per cent.

Although there has only been a gerontological center at Sukhumi for the past seventeen years, the longevity of the Abkhasians
has been systematically studied on several occasions since 1932;
we can thus rely on dates from that time, and there have been instances of people who were even then of great age surviving until
the present day. Only the slightest signs of heart condition were
found in some of the extremely old. A study of their vision showed
that in a group aged over 90, nearly 40 per cent of the men and 30
per cent of the women had vision good enough to thread a needle
without glasses; 40 per cent of the men and women had good
hearing. In addition there were no reported cases of cancer in a
nine-year study of 123 people said to be over 100. They also had
extremely good psychological and neurological stability. Most of
them seemed to have a clear recollection of the past—even the distant past—but of comparatively recent events they knew little, a
characteristic observable among old people of England. In a few
the pattern was reversed, and about 20 per cent retained an equilibrium where this memory of past and present was concerned.

All were able to orientate themselves correctly in regard to time
and space. All showed clear and logical thinking, and the majority
estimated their physical and mental capacities correctly. This logical thinking and correct estimation of their mental capacities is
very important as, for the Abkhasians, unlike the Ecuadorans,
there are no written records (apart from military records: many
of the men served in the army). They showed great interest in the

affairs of their families and they could also give information on historic events in their area—a good method for correlation.

Unlike the Vilcabambans, the Abkhasian women go to a hospital for childbirth. They also have their own highly skilled bonesetters. These are much needed in the community so fond of hunting and riding, where accidents often involve broken limbs. In Ecuador very few have horses; if they ride it is most usually on mule or donkey.

Like the Vilcabambans, they have no time for funerals. If there are any, it is usually only to bury dead children. At Vilcabamba the cemetery is hidden. Among all these communities with centenarians there is a marked lack of interest in the idea of dying, and of death in general. It is as if death was a disease that never happens to them.

The Abkhasians have not always lived on their land. About sixty years ago they were nomadic. As a whole they share Shirali's often-quoted belief that their longevity is due to the tranquillity of the region, the good air, lack of stress and their traditional customs in regard to sex, work and diet. As far as accidents are concerned, there is less fear of them happening in the Soviet Socialist Republic, where the behavior on the roads is much safer than in Ecuador.

The Abkhasians seldom get married until they are thirty and firmly maintain that they do not start sexual relationships until then. Most men retain their sexual potency until long after their seventieth birthday and, in fact, many ninety-year-olds have been shown still to have vigorous sexual relations. Healthy sperm has been taken from these men up to the age of 119. Of the women 13.6 per cent continue to menstruate after the age of fifty-five. In Ecuador, men still father children in their early hundreds, and women may continue to menstruate until their early sixties. Men there marry in their early twenties.

In the fifth century A.D., under Justinian, the Abkhasians became Christians. But in the fifteenth century the area was swept by the Sunni sect of Islam. However, they still have many underlying beliefs that are basically pagan. They still make animal sacrifices at family shrines and there is an element of ancestor worship, which does not seem in the least out of place among such a venerable community. The Abkhasian philosophy of preserving the national culture has been their salvation. Unfortunately, in both Ecuador and Pakistan the trend is toward eliminating the customs of minority groups. Although it could be argued that this is good for national security, it is not particularly good for the communities affected by it, whose daily life and customs are deeply part of their sense of themselves. Radios and television sets are not valued particularly by the Abkhasians; the idea of these machines being conveyers of mass entertainment or instruction has not yet reached them. This could be a reflection on the programs available to them, rather than personal attitudes. Horsemanship is regarded as the most important skill, and a good horseman, of whatever age, is respected throughout the community. They are also keen on fighting, like the Turks—an ethnic group which they greatly resemble.

The men often go into the army, and may not come out of it until they are sixty. After that they often get married, not because they feel that their sexual powers are waning, but because they have led a wandering life and feel that at that age they would like to plan for the future and settle down. The people think of themselves as getting old after reaching one hundred years, or when they can no longer climb trees, or dig the ground in the garden or farm!

There is more content and interest in the lives of the women than we find among the Ecuadoran groups. For example, they are encouraged to look as beautiful as possible and to be able to dance—attributes and accomplishments apparently not valued by the Vilcabambans. In Ecuador, women are seen as little more than sex objects to whom the male applies himself to show how really virile and splendid he is. On one point the two communities, however, agree with regard to women: that the virginity of the girl before marriage is essential. If a man thinks that his wife is not a virgin in Ecuadoran society he can, and will, divorce her at once, and she goes back in disgrace to her parents. In these small communities there will be no chance of marriage for her in these circumstances, so she must leave, usually going to the cities of Quito or Guayaquil. In Abkhasian society the groom has the right to take his erstwhile wife back to her family and to have his marriage gifts returned at the same time, announcing to the family, and to all and sundry: "Take your dead one." In each society the name of the guilty party is demanded, but the girl, often despite everything, and continuing to show spirit, gives the name of someone who has recently died. This avoids a blood feud between the families concerned. Both the Ecuadoran and Russian communities of centenarians were extremely modest in discussing sex: it is rarely talked about and little sexual vulgarity (as we think of it) is seen or heard, at least in public. Extra-marital sex is considered a crime in Ecuador, but in Abkhasian society, within the prescribed boundaries, it is not. This is most probably a reflection of the Roman Catholic and Muslim beliefs.

The extended family plays a great part in the social structure of the Abkhasians and they try to include in it as many relatives, however tenuous the relationship, as they can. The woman, when she marries, goes to the house of her husband and belongs to his family group. The family is also increased by a system of godfathers, who, like our own, attend the "christening" of their godchild, a custom also found in Ecuador.

The majority of the Abkhasians are farmers, and continue to be so until the very end of their days. Those few who have been civil servants, when they retire and leave their jobs generally return to the family farm. Others go on to the collective farm in the locality, where they can work at their own speed under the piecework system.

Dr. Sichinava made a detailed examination of the Abkhasians' work habits. One group included eighty-two men (most of whom were peasants and had been working from the age of eleven) and forty-five women (who from the time of their adolescence had worked in the home and helped in the care of farm animals). He found that the workload decreased considerably between the ages of eighty and ninety for forty-eight of the men, and between ninety and a hundred for the rest. Among the women, twenty-seven of them started doing less work between eighty and ninety while the others started doing less after ninety. The few men who had been shepherds stopped following the herds up to the mountain ledges in the spring, and instead began tending farm animals. After the age of ninety the farmers began to work less land; many stopped plowing and lifting heavy loads, but continued weeding (despite the bending involved) and doing other tasks. Most of the women stopped helping in the fields and some began to do less housework. Instead of serving the entire family—an Abkhasian family which is extended through marriage may include up to sixty people—they started to serve only themselves and their children. But they also leisurely fed the chickens, spun and knitted, as they had been doing for most of their lives.

Dr. Sichinava also observed 21 men and 7 women over 100 years of age and found that, on an average, they worked a four-hour day on the farm. The men weeded and helped to bring in the corn, the women strung the tobacco leaves, a similar work pattern to that of the old women in the villages of centenarians in Ecuador. These people are not slackers; in fact they even have their own work areas. For instance there was Kelkilina Khesa, a woman reputed to be 109 who came from the village of Otapi. One summer she was reputed to have worked 8 hours a day for 49 days. Cozba Basaj, a man of 94 on the same farm, worked 155 days in one given year. At the age of 90, Minosyan Grigorii, from the village of Aragich, worked for 230 days of the year.

The people themselves, and the Russian doctors, declared that their longevity had a strong connection with their working habits. If one does not use a machine, it becomes rusty. If one sits in a chair the whole time, at what is considered to be the end of one's days, the parts are bound to seize up, simply through lack of use. Keeping working and active helps the vital body fluids to circulate, and keeps the muscles toned up and in good condition. The blood supply will then be driven to all parts of the body and, in doing so, it feeds and renews the body cells. The Abkhasians have a particularly apt saying in this context: "Without rest, a man cannot work; without work, the rest does not give you benefit." The old people have learned very skillfully how to alternate rest and work during these days. The piecework system on their farms allows the aged to go along at their own pace. The Abkhasians, as the Ecuadorans, walk a great deal also—another beneficial activity for their health.

As is so often the case outside Western societies, people rarely become fat unless they are ill. Obesity is non-existent among the

working people. Exactly the same situation is found in southern
Ecuador. There was only one person in Vilcabamba who could be
described as obese. All centenarians that I have come across eat
the same food throughout their lives, irrespective of any change in
economic status. Like the centenarian communities of southern
Ecuador, especially those of Vilcabamba, there is among the Abkhasians a great reliance placed on herbal concoctions for cures
of minor ailments, aches and pains, and, some claim, as preventatives against more serious diseases. Both groups have about two
hundred types of herbs that they can call on to benefit their
health. Where the Abkhasians are concerned, it is only after all
the relevant herbal remedies have been tried and found wanting
in any particular case that the orthodox doctor is called in.

Both the Vilcabambans and the Abkhasians produce large
quantities of tobacco. The latter are the main suppliers of tobacco
in the Soviet Union. The Vilcabambans smoke and drink heavily,
which seems to affect them little; the Abkhasians only handle the
weed, but do not smoke it. And, except for some dry red wine
with a low alcohol content, which they have with each meal and
call "life-giving" or "elixir of life," they don't drink at all. They are
very fond of vegetable juices taken as refreshment, and drink
these in much the same way as we drink Coca-Cola. In this respect they are similar to the Hunzucuts (Hunzas) who eat most
of their food accompanied by fresh grape wine.

The Abkhasians eat very little meat—at most twice a week—and
then only in small portions. They prefer chicken, and hate fish.
The meat is boiled very thoroughly, tending to make it rather
tough. With all meals they have abista, a corn meal mash cooked
in salty water, with pieces of homemade goats' milk cheese in it.
They eat cheese daily, and have about two glasses of buttermilk
per day. When they eat eggs, which is no more than twice a week,
they are boiled or fried with cheese, making a kind of welsh rare-
bit.

Fresh fruit and vegetables also play an important part in their
diet. The former are usually grapes and apples, while among the
vegetables are included beans, onions, tomatoes, cucumbers, cabbage, baby lima beans (cooked slowly for many hours, mashed
and flavored with onion sauce, peppers, garlic and pomegranate

juice). There is also a wide variety of pickled vegetables to choose from. As a side dish, there is always a large quantity of garlic, a blood-purifier. Absent from the table is any form of sugar, although honey is taken at times. Thus they have a greater variety of foods than the people of southern Ecuador. The Russian dieticians believe that their intake of buttermilk, pickled vegetables and wine helps to destroy certain harmful bacteria, probably also helping to prevent arteriosclerosis and cancer. The only thing in their diet generally agreed by medical men to be harmful is the hot pepper sauce.

The other community of centenarians that I should like to deal with are the Hunzas or Hunzucuts. They live mainly in northern Pakistan, though there are a few communities in the Sinkiang province of China. The two groups are separated as a result of a political division—the boundary between northern Pakistan and China runs right through their territory. Little is known about the group of the Hunzas in Sinkiang, but those of northern Pakistan are about thirty thousand in number. They live in the area northeast of the Khyber Pass, where there is also a common border with Russia, close to the third highest peak in the world, Mount Rakaposhi. Among the most recent visitors to these people are Lowell Thomas in 1957, and Alan E. Banik in 1958. Renee Taylor accompanied the latter, and returned to the area in the early 1960s. They reported that many of the Hunzucut males lived to the ages of 120 and 140, but there are no reliable statistics to back this up and no one has been able to research into these people properly, least of all since the early 1960s for political reasons.

The Hunzas live in a similar setting to that of Vilcabamba. The only way to reach the town nearby is by air from Gilgit. Progress up to the Hunza valley depends upon the weather, and landslides are not infrequent.

They are a white-skinned people, like the majority of Vilcabambans. Legends say that they are the descendants of some soldiers of Alexander and his Persian consorts. Their villages are on the route through to China (Sinkiang) (as the Vilcabambans are on the route to Peru). The community is divided socially into three sections: the young years (up to thirty years), the middle years (thirty to sixty years) and the "rich" years (sixty and over). As in Abkhasia and Ecuador, the people don't retire from working. They exercise a great deal, working on the farm and walking to the village. Unlike the Vilcabambans, they have no childhood diseases such as mumps, measles, chicken pox; later in life they have no ulcers, except occasionally those caused by hepatitis.

Animals are scarce, this time owing to the limitation of land. For the mountains rise sheer almost from the edge of the valley, and this limits their fields. These are carefully tended, giving them mineral manures and compost. They say that what they take out they must put back in another form. They live on indigenous foods from their small holdings, and for them the care of their land comes before everything. They themselves think that the water, which contains much iron, copper, calcium and fluoride, is the secret of their excellent health.

The diet of the Hunzas is grain and pulse-based, as with the Ecuadorans. This includes wheat, barley and buckwheat, Job's-tears (a large seed used as a grain) and small grains. Green vegetables such as spinach and lettuce, root vegetables such as carrots, turnips, potatoes and radishes, are eaten. Beans, chickpeas and other pulses such as lentils and sprouted pulses are part of their diet, and they also eat marrows and pumpkins, as well as plenty of cottage cheese; herbs are used in tea and for seasoning (as with the Ecuadorans and Abkhasians).

Their fruits are chiefly wild apricots and wild mulberries, eaten fresh or sun-dried. The stones of the apricots are cracked for the kernels. Other fruit are usually eaten raw; there is little fuel around to boil them—when they are cooked it is more like steaming. This shortage of cooking facilities may be one reason why they eat so little meat—meat is eaten only on rare occasions. The lack of meat-eating in the case of the Ecuadorans is because of poverty.

They drink plenty of spring water, with which they are amply supplied; also fresh wine, like the Russian centenarians. It is generally not drunk before it is ninety days old, and is not kept for very long after this. They also drink fresh goats' milk, buttermilk (*lassi*) and clarified butter.

13

Our Discoveries— and the Genetic and Environmental Arguments

Longevity is thought by some geneticists to run in families—rather like baldness. There are a lot of arguments in favor of this, and many examples of long-lived families. In the majority of the instances of the long-lived people to be found in Britain, this longevity does tend to run in their families. Their members sometimes survive in spite of an apparently unfortunate environment. Thus, many of the people that we see lingering on in old people's homes until they are 110 or 112 probably have their family tree to thank for their length of life. Often, however, these people have lost many of their faculties, which does not make living to a great age appealing.

Both the genetic and the environmental approach to longevity are of great importance. Individual, isolated cases of centenarians present different evidence from whole communities of them; it seems natural in the latter case at least to pursue environmental factors as being possible causes or contributory factors to longevity.

The geneticists interested in longevity have thought that there must have been some strain of longevity in the Spaniards who settled in Ecuador. As they were Spaniards, they did not wish to breed with the local Indians, and kept a very inbred community. Too many of these geneticists have taken the genetic basis for granted, without investigating sufficiently. There are many families involved in the area; they could, in fact, just as well belong to the remnants of some ancient white race, which remained by the grace of the conquistadores. The lucidity and the alertness of these supercentenarians is not necessarily accounted for by genetics. But some researchers have not considered the environmental effect as significant.

The five communities we visited in Ecuador were of no one racial type; inbreeding was very unlikely. La Toma, for instance, has a population with no traceable ancestry—they are a hotchpotch, living on the crossroads of the main road to Peru. Many people stop here, and students from Loja and the coastal towns visit it at weekends, sowing their wild oats. I think no one would claim that the forebears of these villagers could be traced back easily to a single racial group! And yet these are communities with a high population of centenarians. The other areas we visited did not have a centenarian population of a single racial type either.

The attitude that environment can be ignored as a cause seems to defeat the very purpose of science. These places should at least be studied before judgments on environment are made, for the people are, as we all are, the creatures of their environment, as well as of their genetic inheritance.

There has been a considerable amount of laboratory study, on mice and rats, to assess the effect of diet on longevity. Sir Robert Macarrison, one of the world's leading nutritionists, spent many years in India and among the Hunzas. He built up a fine library, which is now with Dr. Hugh Sinclair, of Magdalen College, Oxford. As a result of his many years of association with India, including seven years among the Hunzas, he became an expert on the diet of that region. When he returned to his country he continued with experiments and research into diet, and did much work on rats in this respect, as the following examples will show.

He took twelve hundred rats and fed them for twenty-seven months (equivalent, it is estimated, to fifty years in human terms), on a mainly Hunza diet; this consisted of chapatis made of whole-meal flour, lightly smeared with fresh butter. He also gave them sprouted pulses, fresh raw carrots, wild apricots, and a small ration of meat with bone once a week. They drank unboiled milk and an abundance of water. None of these rats became ill and, in fact, they all died a natural death at an old age.

He next tried this diet on the survivors of a thousand rats previously fed on the typical diet of the Indians of the Central Plains, as a result of which they had developed various diseases; almost immediately their symptoms of malnutrition began to improve, and they survived to a ripe old age.

From his researches Macarrison also found out that the fewer calories rats were given the longer they lived. His studies were applied to humans, and his experiments on diet formed an important basis for dietetic theory, which has gradually become more and more prominent both among laymen and medical men—that a correct diet can prolong life.

The communities where centenarians are found have in common their diet, which is frugal, low in calories and closely linked to the soil, from which most of the food they eat is taken direct. This connection with the soil is a very important factor, as it relates to important discoveries we made about the trace elements in the soil in Ecuador. These, we feel, are a crucial element in environmental factors contributing to longevity. Clearly, as Macarrison's researches and our own show, the calorie content of diet, and its composition, is a significant factor in health and aging.

In the 1940s caloric restriction was first studied in laboratory tests; it was supposed that this would slow down the aging processes, in many species from insects to rats; and it was effective. In these studies young animals were half starved, and kept in a juvenile condition, until all the other fully fed rats in the group of equal age were senile. If those that had been starved were then well fed, most started to grow and develop, and live, on average, a great deal longer than their well-fed contemporaries.

After much experimentation, it was found that rodents fed on 60 per cent of their normal calorie intake, but in all other respects normally, had a 40 per cent longer life-span than the control group, fed on a normal diet. The method was to feed normally for two days out of three. In the animals that were experimented on, not only was the first group's life prolonged, but all the usual

diseases, including tumors, were held in check. So far, in gerontological studies in the laboratory, this has been the greatest leap
forward.

What else has been discovered? Scientists have found out that if
711 male mice are fed with a certain amount of anti-oxidants
(chemicals, blackish-looking in color, that are put into vegetable
oils and rubber as preservatives in commerce—a natural anti-ox-
idant is vitamin E) in their mash, they live longer, 100 days longer
in fact, than the control mice. The average life-span of a laboratory male mouse is 551.6 days, but if given anti-oxidants they can
live to an average of 651.5 days, some being so strong that they
can live 900 days. Female mice have a slightly shorter expectation
of life than their male partners.

There are other tests being carried out on mice now. Tests are
being made of substances that stimulate the liver (a well-known
substance of this type is DDT, and there are indications that this
can prolong life; there are other similar effects). Trace elements
and poisons, such as arsenic, and even the American Indian's
deadly curare, can be beneficial in small doses. These are thought
to act by spoiling the appetite, thus keeping the animal in a half-
starved condition. But in the Third World there are many people
in a condition of half-starvation and the only thing this seems to
do is to help shorten the life. Presumably a low-calorie but *selec-
tive* diet is a possible answer.

Dietary experiments are important, and as yet the factors
affected by diet are only speculative—cell generation, stress symptoms, waste products, diminishment of the effects of obesity. It is
believed that a suitable diet could increase the period of adult
vigor by 20 per cent, depending, of course, upon what age it was
started.

One of the problems of these experiments is that they have been
on mice, and so far it is not known how applicable they would be
to humans. In the large areas of malnutrition and low-calorie diets
of the world, few people show signs of longevity. In fact, often the
opposite is seen; people in these areas can look seventy when they
are only forty, and the expectation of life is very low in such communities. Yet obviously diets with too many calories are equally
bad for health.

Let us here, having stated the unquestionable importance of hereditary factors in longevity and discussed some of the laboratory experiments on animals in this field, summarize the factors we studied in the centenarians of Ecuador.

In our investigation of environmental factors possibly accounting for, or contributory to, longevity, we felt that undoubtedly the most exciting and significant single factor was the trace elements found in the soil, water and diet. This is not to say that we think they alone account for longevity. But they are significant, and worth emphasizing.

Samples of water and soil were taken from the valleys in and near the "crescent." We discovered from our analyses of these that the water was very pure, having hardly any minerals in it. The soil, on the other hand, is full of minerals, which are not soluble in water. It was found to contain a good deal of gold (which has been mined here for many generations), large quantities of iron, and, most importantly, large quantities of magnesium and cadmium, both comparatively rare trace elements. The centenarians all live surrounded by high mountains, so that the trace elements are leached off the higher ground in some quantities and deposited in the valleys. Now it is known that trace elements are able to pass from the soil into foodstuffs—i.e. one finds trace elements in seeds, etc.

The effects of trace elements on bodily health and function are significant, as may be the interplay of various trace elements upon each other. Certainly it is true that there was a marked pinkish coloration of the soil where we found these pockets of longevity. And the striking and extreme tooth decay found among these people may well be connected with the action of rare trace elements— and the fact that longevity and this unusual tooth decay exist side by side is fascinating. It may lead us to some important conclusions. This tooth condition has existed since pre-Colombian times, as can be seen from some of the skulls I was shown. Since working in this area, I have discussed the problem of trace elements with several scientists, and believe that it is possible there is some rare trace element reaction; only by the continued study of the geobotany of this area could this be conclusively verified. Meanwhile, these trace elements are an exciting discovery, to be pursued even further.

Apart from this rather dramatic discovery, we studied other factors, and found some more significant than others. A crucial factor was that the oldest inhabitants were in fact those living outside the villages, and thus living a different life, and eating very different food, healthier in content and lower in calories. As we know, diet and health are closely connected, and thus the significance of these mountain small holdings and their way of life, unaffected by the towns and town food, is something we take very seriously.

These are some of our other conclusions:

Altitude. Among the "islands of longevity" throughout the world there seems to be a common factor. This is a certain altitude. In Ecuador, Vilcabamba, Nambacola, La Toma, San Pedro and, in the north, Ambuki, are all in valleys at about a height of seventeen hundred to nineteen hundred meters. This is about the same height as the Lietschental valley in Switzerland, the Caucasus, and the Hunzas valley on the Pakistan/China borders.

Aridity of the areas. The regions in Ecuador where communities of centenarians have been found have a very low rainfall, Vilcabamba having the highest. Generally they are very dry and dusty. This is very much in keeping with the other regions of the world where centenarians are to be found.

The Equator. Many people, especially the Ecuadorans, believe that behind the longevity of the centenarians is the fact of their being on the Equator, and that this gives them balance, in temperament and bodily cells. The chief advocate of this idea is Dr. J. Lovewisdom, an American doctor who can show sixteen certificates of doctorates, who has lived in Vilcabamba valley for several years. But this theory has no scientific foundation, especially if we consider the communities of centenarians in the rest of the world, in most cases quite far removed from the Equator. Dr. Synge, the man who discovered amino acids and who is a Nobel peace prize winner, holds that in certain areas near the Equator are found remarkable qualities in plants. And Magnus Pike, the director of the British Association for the Advancement of Science, agrees with Dr. Synge in this respect. The Russians are at present working on these theories in their research establishments.

Diet. This may be a powerful contributory factor, and, until recently, I thought that it was the main factor in longevity. Ecuadorans consume fewer calories (in fact, half that of the average Englishman) than is customary in the Western world. However, this is true of a large percentage of the world's population, especially in the Third World, yet we only find centenarians in clearly defined areas. This seems to indicate that longevity can at best only be affected in part by diet. I think that Professor Leaf of Harvard University agrees with this view. Nevertheless, the mountain diet is the basis for other attributes—such as their fitness and lack of obesity; their good health, at least indirectly, and their long life.

Drink. Ecuadorans have a habit of drinking large amounts of liquor. Usually they drink from four to six cupfuls daily; often it is up to a bottle per day, to quite old age. In this way they have, at least, discovered a form of relaxation. But the women do not drink, and perhaps one of the contributory factors to their dying younger may be that they thus have no escape valve. Abkhasians and Hunzas also consume a considerable amount of drink. This has led some to believe that consumption of alcohol helps prolong their lives. The theory has no scientific backing.

Ethnic origins. There is a theory among Vilcabambans that the centenarian inhabitants of this valley are the descendants of an ethnic group dating back to pre-Colombian times. Evidence comes from the skin, oval heads, enormous beaked noses and remarkably large ears of the centenarians, for they are remarkably similar to the heads depicted on pieces of ceramic dating back fifteen hundred years or more and found in the Andean regions of South America. These people, it is supposed, made overtures at the time of the Conquest, which were accepted, took Spanish names for protection, or were ignored, and survived because of their geographical isolation. Thus it is thought that their great age has a mainly genetic basis.

This is an intriguing idea, but it does not hold water when we take the recently discovered villages into consideration; *their* inhabitants are made up of Mestizos, Spanish, Creoles (from the coast) and Indian stock, and, if we are to include Ambuki, Negro stock. Equally, the idea popular among the Lojans and some American scientists that the inhabitants, at least of Vilcabamba, are descended from Spanish soldiers who retreated to the isolated area after the Spanish defeat at the battle of Pichincha in 1825 does not support a genetic hypothesis—for there is no reason to believe that the Spanish soldiers involved in this were, by some peculiar trick of fate, from the longest living families in Spain, as they would have to be if the ethnic group argument is to be upheld.

Genetic factors. It is widely believed at present that longevity in Ecuador runs in families. Some believe that years ago a group of centenarians banded themselves together and decided that they would live all their days in Vilcabamba—the Sacred Valley. Again, it is believed that, by a process of natural selection over the years, the people who lived long survived, while the others died out. At the moment there is a strong lobby for the genetic argument, and that these groups are all intermarried. So far this has been very difficult to establish, especially as so many people in a village have the same name.

Sex linkage. Generally it has been found that the very oldest people in the world, i.e. those over 110, are male. Then come spinster females; it is supposed that the lack of stress in their lives is an aid to longevity especially the lack of the hazards of child-bearing.

Sleep. The majority of the communities where we find the centenarians throughout the world live in technologically primitive areas. They go to bed with the sun and get up with the sun, to a degree unknown in developed parts of the world. Those that are living on the Equator, or near the equatorial line, therefore have much the same amount of sleep each day of the year. This regularity may aid their longevity, whether by accident or not. They have few clocks or radios to let them know the time of the day, and depend almost entirely on their observations of the sun's movements. Many doctors believe that this regular sleep pattern is an aid to longevity, especially in Western countries. Western centenarians rarely suffer from insomnia. Many people have asked me, when discussing the centenarians of the Andes, if they sleep much of their lives away, and this is so—about half their lives are spent sleeping.

Plants and herbs. There are numerous herbs used in a variety of ways in these areas of Ecuador—mainly by the older generations. One of these in particular seems to have the remarkable effect of preventing and helping to cure cancer. This is the condurango. It is a plant somewhat similar to ivy, the bark being poisonous. This must certainly be studied further. Other herbs act as stimulants, astringents, depressants or narcotics. Guayuna, a narcotic and a member of the holly family, is used to improve the fertility of women and the virility of males. Incidentally, it is an interesting point that sea holly roots were used in "comfits," as an aphrodisiac in Elizabethan times. Matico is also used in the treatment of kidney and liver ailments; it is a depressant, and a member of the pepper family.

From cedron and the bark of the cascarilla tree (the cinchona variety) are made health-giving teas. Cascarilla is a member of the quinine group of trees, and it has the same properties. The old name for it is Peruvian bark. It was first found at Malacatos by the Jesuits, and much used. A worldwide trade grew up for the quinine obtained from it, since for hundreds of years quinine was the only known cure for malaria. The fruit of the spiny cactus (tuna) was considered a great delicacy, with health-giving properties. Many serious diseases are thought to be traceable to impurities in the blood—and cedron is known to act as a great blood-purifier.

There are many other kinds of herbs used for anything from the improvement of the hair to that of the heart. But none of these herbs are considered to have rejuvenating properties—they are considered rather as cures for various diseases and conditions. It is possible that in this way they help survival.

The only plant that I have known to be sought after to rejuvenate is the soma plant of India, mentioned by Sushruta, the famous surgeon/physician of the Indian Middle Ages. One concoction of the soma root was eaten, another was used to bathe in, and, according to accounts, in seven weeks the patient was completely rejuvenated. There are, of course, many legends about rejuvenation—like the one among the Italians that living solely on grapes helps people live longer.

The wilco. This tree is found throughout the West Indies and the northern part of South America, under a variety of names such as aculpa, doda and job, all bearing no resemblance to the name that it has in the vicinity of Vilcabamba. Its seeds are used by shamans for creating trances and comas. None of its remarkable properties are thought to prolong age. By some it is considered a tree with sacred properties, and the reason why the valley of Vilcabamba was so named. The tree is in no way peculiar to the valley—it is very widespread. Its seeds are a kind of cure-all, and, above all, are regarded as important for their trance-inducing qualities.

Lack of stress. At times of stress the males drink themselves into a stupor; they also do this regularly on weekends. The women show more signs of stress, looking much older for their years, and they don't live so long.

The people of the valleys are calm by nature, and, living usually in such isolated places, there is little to cause stress. However, some of the oldest people we found almost seem to court stress e.g. Castillo Calderon (116) of La Chonta, near Nambacola, goes by bus to the coast. This entails a two-hour walk from his farm to the bus stop, followed by a twelve-hour bus journey—an ordeal that he must face again on the return journey. There is thus some indication that it is *prolonged* stress which kills or harms the human metabolism.

14

Conclusions—and the
Future of the Villages

Scientists interested in longevity are agreed that, because of their authenticated birth certificates, the Ecuadoran centenarians are by far the most significant of all groups. These are the blueprints for any study in depth of centenarians. The hundreds of certificates that we saw are undoubtedly genuine and can be seen by anyone wishing to investigate further. Many of them are in sheepskin registers. On their first few pages is combined information on births and deaths, starting, in the case of Gonzanamá, in 1655. In the case of San Pedro, the records go back to 1770. Those of Vilcabamba only go back to 1852. We have to go to Malacatos for anything earlier.

These are all ecclesiastical records. Civil record books began to be established in 1902 in the villages. These are often much larger books, and clothbound. In some cases they give more information than the ecclesiastical records—the cause of a person's death, e.g. accident, influenza, or, in the case of children, measles, gastroenteritis etc. This information could be made an important study in itself. Cases of cancer and heart ailments are conspicuous by their absence; what the people themselves say, that they do not get these ailments, is borne out by these records.

The people we studied do not have the same pattern of sicknesses as we do—diseases common to us, such as cancer and diabetes, are almost unknown. Yet in the surrounding areas, where no centenarians are found, these same diseases are quite common.

The Vilcabambans do not excel in vigor in their middle years, but they keep what vigor they have for a far greater life-span than anyone else in the world—including the villagers in the rest of southern Ecuador. But if one wants to see people who are strikingly vigorous throughout their lives, one must go to San Pedro de la Bendita. They have a greater general vitality than anyone else that I have come across, especially as a group.

Though we may need blueprints if we are to build a house, it is just as essential to have bricks for the final results. So it is with the human body. Thus we should regard as blueprints the chromosomes and the environmental factors as the bricks involved in the building. There has been and is, where human beings are concerned, too much neglect of these bricks and their study.

The centenarians of the sierras of Ecuador all live in a region and in a manner that have certain things in common. In addition, at least four ethnic groups are found among these old people. In some cases the groups have not been very long in their valleys, e.g. San Pedro and Ambuki. Therefore, to study their environment for an answer to the riddle of longevity is crucial, rather than repeated backward assertions about their genetic development. We see that nearly all centenarians are closely involved with the land in their lives and the bulk of their food is grown in the locality.

In England, districts play an important part in the pattern of age and disease. For instance, cancer of the stomach is found most commonly in northern Wales. The oldest people are to be found living along the coast of East Anglia, Norfolk, and the coastal areas of south Devon. Recently, I have been looking into the possible reasons for the great ages reached by some people living along the coast of Norfolk. These people do not have a very easy life, especially in winter. Again, the majority for the greater part of their lives obtained most of their food from their large gardens, and from the locality. They thought a possible cause of their great ages was living mainly upon fresh fruit and vegetables. If we take an over-all look at England, we find that those people who are working in agriculture live the longest, followed closely by clergymen; then come amateur naturalists. These groups also have the lowest incidence of cancer. Most are thought to have a capacity to relax; they are also less surrounded by polluted air. Also, at least until recently, these three groups were not noted for their wealth, and could not afford rich food—plain food was the order of the day.

Those people who are happy in their work, whatever it may be, look younger for their ages, probably because they lack tension. We have only to look at the papers over a few years to see which are the groups who tend to die early: film stars, who live a life of stress, are followed, as the statistics show, by lawyers, newsmen and bus conductors, who also have lives of tension (and, where the two latter groups are concerned, great physical unrest as well —snatching at meals here and there whenever they have an odd moment). People in these jobs often suffer from ulcers and cancer, cancer of the stomach being the most common type, as it is generally for the male in England.

From what Dr. J. Santiana, the cancer expert in Quito, told me, there was a similar pattern in the big towns of Ecuador, Quito, Cuenca and Guayaquil. In these cities, much of the Western diet has been adopted for a number of years. Butter and other saturated fats are now eaten, as is meat. They have many cases of heart conditions in these cities also. The cholesterol level in the centenarians we studied was strikingly low.

Most of the scientists who have shown an interest in these centenarians and their longevity seem already half-convinced that the centenarians are an end product of some isolated group of people who have built up some strange resistance over many thousands of years (though how this can be so when most scientists believe that man has only been in South America for eight thousand years is hard to see). They find it difficult to comprehend that there are different racial groups involved.

Also I suspect that the possibility of looking into their environment seems far too simple for some scientists; there is less room for complicated intellectual argument, which seems to be the main ingredient necessary to warrant the beginning of vast projects involving many thousands of pounds and animals' lives—and which often end quite inconclusively.

This study will at least show that if more work was done on the environment of human beings directly, and with success, the pursuit of many animal experiments would be unnecessary and incomplete—i.e. genetics cannot explain everything, but we do need to know how people live and the factors in their lives and surroundings which affect them mentally and physically. For such studies, as ours has shown, could bear rich results in telling us more about the mysterious similarities and differences among peoples the world over. These centenarians bear dramatic witness to many psychological and philosophical attitudes and theories of old age, and we have much still to learn from them.

What of the future of these regions? There are many superlatives in South America, with its snow-capped mountains, strange animals and exotic plant life. The inhabitants are used to what is, to us, the unusual. The views in these valleys can have changed little in the last two thousand years, though they may have changed color, for what is now a brown distance was, in days gone by, a green one. Though there have been some very bad earthquakes and landslides, they would not have changed the landscape to any great extent. All the places that I mention in this book where the centenarians live are in no way shut in by the mountains—they are in spacious, open country or spreading out from the foot of mountains, and always at an altitude of seventeen hundred to nineteen hundred meters. Most of the changes that have come about are due to the activities of man—burning off the undergrowth, cutting down trees and hedgerows for sugar cane, clearing land for a growing population.

The whole region is a place of unique botanical interest, and a richness not found elsewhere. It is a geo-botanist's paradise! There would be much value in a research station at Vilcabamba to look at the plant life. It is unfortunate that these places are being discovered only on the *edge* of a medicinal era that is beginning again to attach importance to substances obtained from plants and information obtained from folklore. The past favored the centenarian. It is only since new kinds of adulterated foods have penetrated into these villages that the diet has changed—a diet not beneficial to health or longevity, as can be seen from the local towns. From what the centenarians tell us about the plants that they used to collect, much reliance was placed on herbs to augment the mainstay foods such as maize and the potato, and to make them more appetizing.

As for the study and preservation of various plants for cures and other uses, it has been the Medical Research Council that has been the most aware. It was Dr. Conrad Gorinsky of St. Bartholomew's Hospital Medical School who, with a grant from the MRC, managed to save the recipe and to obtain the curare poison from the South American Indians (who are now dying out). This is now a vital factor, used in small doses, in the cure of some heart conditions previously thought hopeless. Other bodies that one would naturally look to, such as the World Health Organization, have not yet become very involved in these matters. At the moment they act, for the most part, as a post office for the various medical groups throughout the world.

There is little machinery in the big foundations for the allocation of grants for the study of useful medicinal plants such as the condurango, which is thought to be a cure for cancer. This is bound to come, however, in a decade or so, but will this be too late? One would hope that these plants will at least be preserved, for they are only found in a few valleys, and their value may be great. But already they are being eradicated in Ecuador to make more land available for sugar cane.

The destruction of the valleys has been great, and still continues, with badly made roads being built in the region, the continued chopping down of trees, the destruction of hedges to make use of every inch of the rich soil, which seems to contain every suitable ingredient to make crops flourish. Luckily, Vilcabamba has some water meadows and these, at the moment, are a reserve for the precious herbs and plants. But these, too, are now being threatened with drainage, so that yet more sugar cane can be planted. Many of the mountain areas are bare, and the next stage of destruction could be wind erosion—from the gentle cooling breeze that blows from 12:00 to 3:00 P.M. each day, coming from the mountains. It could sweep the top soil off, leaving the area around the village a dusty place, as has occurred elsewhere in South America. The village needs preserving, but in such a way as to ensure the preservation of the many positive and rare factors in the area.

Shortly after I arrived there in 1974, I was asked to make a plan and offer suggestions for the building of a sanatorium at Vilcabamba. I feel that a sanatorium by itself would do little good except to exploit the villagers and benefit big business. Therefore I suggested a plan whereby the project would be part sanatorium, part research laboratory, so that not only the sick people could be studied but also the other people of the area, their diet and their whole environment. A few days later two men from a large Ecuadoran company came to visit me wanting to hear my ideas. It would be difficult, but vital, to ensure that the villagers reaped at least some of the benefit of such a plan; that, for instance, when the sanatorium was being built, pipes should be taken to the houses of the village with full sanitary arrangements. The sanatorium would have to be part of a complete scheme, embracing the whole of the village.

In the laboratory samples of plants could also be studied, and soil and water samples, to pursue our own discoveries on the importance of trace elements, etc. Such a center would be ideal, and workers there could report their findings to other such centers abroad.

However, there are many difficulties here: who would administer the funds, and where would the center be? There are many local problems of administration too. The true cost of the land around would rocket, and make it impossible for future Vilcabambans to live there; the villagers might be told to leave to make way for a government hotel (this has been mentioned—at the moment only in passing—but the idea is already there). All this would be disruptive and destructive to the life of the area.

Would the other "centenarian" villages also be included? If the people who administered the money and the center were in Loja, big business would flourish, large roads would be built to the center, and the goose that laid the golden egg would be destroyed under a mass of tourists, without the scientists having had a chance of investigating these supercentenarians. The people who have already bought land in the vicinity of Vilcabamba would not like to see any rival villages of similar type flourish, and when the top men of the province have investments in the area it is very difficult to suggest other places. Many people hated to see the arrival of big business interests to take over Vilcabamba—especially as big business was connected with the local hospital, which had a very bad record of deaths, and was very backward. On the other hand, if the central government, at Quito, administered the center, it would be too remote to understand all the local conditions and activities.

One answer would be an outside group coming in and taking care of the future of the valleys. It could be put in the care of WHO; but many of the local people would naturally hate this. Whatever is done, it will have to be done soon if these few villages are to survive in a condition that will enable the scientist and the doctor to make a full and unbiased study, for the benefit of all mankind.

These valleys have all the ingredients for development: with good irrigation they would be highly fertile. With the planting of more flowers, herbs and trees, and more good water brought to them, they could probably return to what they must once have looked like, before they were raped along with the rest of the land around. The land has been exploited, then left, and the people responsible have flocked to the cities.

The present main village of Vilcabamba is not the first. There are indications of three previous villages. On the mountains above the villages are found crude hut circles that would have belonged to primitive tribes early on—probably nomadic. Again, there are extensive ruins of a town, or large community, in a craterlike depression on the peak of Lambomuna mountain; in fact this could be the site of a very early settlement. The villages of the southern complex are well grouped together—that is within sixty miles of each other: a region well defined, and not impossible to reach, where, at the moment, and probably for some time to come, the people are eager and interested in any project that may get started. What about the dangers of sensational tourism? How long would the region remain tolerable for the locals and useful for scientists? In a year, most people would be bored by the findings, people would start to question the authenticity, and soon it would be lost to science. The project has to be carefully handled.

The local people in these villages must not be exploited, whatever the nature of the eventual project—this is vital. They are unlikely to be hostile to something which takes their own welfare as paramount. The project should be formulated at a national level, and private local people must not be allowed to exploit the area. It should be similar to that in the Galapagos Islands, with which scientists have already had much useful experience. A group of doctors and scientists, geneticists, environmentalists, and others should be part of the project, and though tourists should not be entirely excluded—indeed this would be virtually impossible—tourism should be controlled so that it does not impair the lives of the locals, or the crucial work of the doctors and scientists.

Gerontology is a comparatively new field, and here is an opportunity to bring the laboratory into the field. Aging in man is so complex, and takes so long; the conditions of environment are very important, and we must not lose this chance to explore them. If the "islands of longevity" can survive another ten years or so, then I would consider them safe—that is, if the existing new enlightenment continues. But they should be saved for posterity. If these old people disappear without our finding some of their secrets, it will be one of the greatest losses to mankind in the history of medical research. Geneticists and environmentalists should work together to discover the secrets of old age—and these people of Ecuador offer us a unique opportunity. We must grasp it.

Index

Abaca, Pastos, 67
Abarca, María, 48
Abkhasians, *xiii*, 16, 113, 114–17, 118, *map*, 111; age, 113; appearance, 113; authenticity, 105, 112–13; community relationship, 116; comparative study, 110–23; drinking, 131; food, 122; health, 114, 115, 118, 121; housing, 114; lifestyle, 113–16; location, 113; marriage, 119–20; number, 110; occupations, 113, 120; records, 117; religion, 110, 114, 118–19; social structure, 116; stature, 116; wealth, 112, 115
Academicians, *xiv*
Accidents, 67, 69, 118
Acosta-Solis, Dr., 12–13, 14
Affluence, 60, 137
Africa, 75
Age-consciousness, 4
Aged, the: attitudes toward, *xiii*, 1–5, 106, 108; death, 99; genetics, 69; loss of faculties, 125; oldest recorded people, 81; percentage of population, 100–1, 117; psychology, 116; quality of life, 69–70; security, 116; value, 4; West, 69. *See* Centenarians
"Age-known specimens," 52
Aging, *xii*; affects, 47; diet, 127; factors, *xii*, *xiii* (*see under* type); mystery, *xiii*, 4; prevention, 66 (*see* Gerontology)
Agriculture, 28, 30, 32–34, 41, 64, 65, 80, 84, 88, 90, 91, 92–96, 107, 115, 124; coffee, 33–34; collective farms, 120; longevity, 137; sugar, 34, 92, 139; system, 90, 92–93

Aguirre, Dolores, 67
Aguirre, Ricardo, 73, 74
Aimpa (herb), 66
Alexander the Great, 123
Altitude, 6–7, 39, 67, 77, 79, 81, 101, 130, 138; aging factor, *xiv*; "islands of longevity," 130
Amazon Basin, 19
Ambuki district, 7, 80, 81, 130, 131, 136
Ancestor worship, 118–19
Andes, 6, 8, 67, 106
Animals, 34–35, 39, 40, 45, 48, 61–62, 65, 76, 84, 89–90, 92–94 ff., 98, 124; diet, 102; experiments, 138; parallel study, 102; philosophy toward, 39; sacrifices, 118–19
Anthropologists, 8, 110, 117
Anthropomorphism, 7
Aphrodisiacs, 133
Arabia, *xiv*
Aragich (village), 121
Archaeology, 8–9, 39, 51
Architecture, 85
Atahualpa, King, 22, 36–37, 79; murder, 37
Atmosphere, 28–29, 35, 39
Australia: Tasmanians, *xi*
Azerbaijan, 113

Baby sitters, 4
Baku, 113
Banik, Alan E., 123
Baptismal certificates, 101, 104, 105
Barzavu (village), 113
Basaj, Cozba, 121
Benet, Sula, 117
Bering Straits landbridge, 8
Birds, 58, 89, 95, 98